Praise for

On Eagle's Wings

What a moving story! Annie's passion for life and her ability to turn obstacles into great opportunities is truly inspiring and will make you want to examine your life to make it better. The impact Annie had on everyone she met is beautifully written in *On Eagle's Wings,* and her story is a testament to her faith, fortitude, and passion for life.

As the Founder of Great Comebacks, I have read thousands of stories but none more powerful than Annie's. She was a beautiful lady who touched everyone she met and whose grace and faith are an inspiration to all of us.

—**Rolf Benirschke,** former placekicker for the
San Diego Chargers, spokesman for the Crohn's and
Colitis Foundation of America, and founder of
Great Comebacks, an IBD patient advocacy program

Despite decades of unrelenting pain and debilitation, Annie Stites was the life-affirming embodiment of the "miracle baby," a name bestowed on her shortly after her birth and first surgery. Stites' determination to triumph over her countless episodes of illness was in no small part motivated by her dedication to offering people and animals her enormous compassion and support, as a friend and teacher. Parker repays the gift of Annie's friendship by sharing her journals' movingly evocative prose, crafting a biography filled with warmth, insight, and love, an inspiring antidote to the cruel illness Stites battled. As Stites wrote, "You are not in control of your physical body, but you can make a choice."

—**Jon Reiner,** James Beard Foundation
Award-winning author of *The Man Who Couldn't Eat*

Almost all patients with Crohn's disease will require an operation within their lifetimes. The magnitude of these operations varies from simple drainage of a subcutaneous abscess to a major intestinal resection with or without an ostomy. As a rule, the younger the patient is at the onset of Crohn's disease, the greater the number of surgeries he or she will require. The greater the number of operations a patient undergoes, the greater the technical difficulty and potential for adverse clinical outcome.

I performed quite a few of Annie's twenty-eight surgeries over the course of her lifetime. As I reflect on my surgical care of Annie over the years, I don't believe I have ever witnessed more consistent and repeated examples of courage. This courage was most evident during her postoperative recoveries and is perhaps best expressed in her own words: "How you deal with disease or this surgery is a matter of choice. You can choose to be depressed and defeated, or you can pick up your head and look around you to all the support of your family and friends, and hang on to that love like a lifeline, for indeed it is."

Long ago I concluded that an important goal of this journey we call life is to try to make a difference in the world. Annie Stites made many differences in the world, including making me a wiser surgeon and more empathetic caregiver.

—**John L. Rombeau, M.D.**, Annie's surgeon

WARNING: ANNIE STITES IS CONTAGIOUS! Do not read this book unless you are willing to be infected by her irrepressible love of life, humanity, and nature. She will cartwheel off these pages into your heart, and you will fall in love. You will know Annie as a patient, whose chronic Crohn's disease tested but never defeated her determination not only to live, but to thrive. Gail Parker has offered us a gift of immeasurable value—Annie. Receive this gift at your own risk. Be prepared to laugh, cry, and be awestruck by this remarkable woman. You've been warned.

—**Dr. John McClay,** retired psychologist, professor, and author

Annie had the uncanny ability to transcend her own unfathomable pain to seek the very best possible outcomes and live life to the fullest. Annie's great empathy was reflected in her unconditional love of all living things—particularly of her dear animals that had some specific deficit. Thank you, Ms. Parker, for allowing us to catch a glimpse of Annie's life with such sensitivity and compassion.

—**Linda J. Heller, Esq.,** award-winning special education advocate

Annie is a rare, delightful, inspirational person who overcomes tremendous personal life odds for happiness that is contagious to everyone around her. This book will make you a happier person.

—**Raymond E. Tobey, M.D.,** former professor of anesthesiology and medical researcher

On Eagle's Wings describes how a positive attitude and a whole lot of grit can allow one to rise above the circumstances of a devastating disease. Annie found escape and adventure on the open water in their sailboat *Freyja*. As a sailor, I can understand how the wonders and challenges of sailing can override other mental and physical demands. *On Eagle's Wings* is an engaging read and an inspiration.

—**Ralph E. Stephens, Ph.D.,** molecular biology researcher with over one hundred scientific publications

Gail Parker's words are beautifully interwoven with journal entries from her sister-in-law, Annie. *On Eagle's Wings* is an all-inspiring book about Annie's faith-driven and triumphant attitude of kicking the odds with a debilitating disease. It is a chronicle of Annie's voracious ability to remain positive after a multitude of surgeries and of her undying love and loyalty to a life well lived!

—**Stacey P. Morgan,** author of *AlphaPET Zoup A to Z,*
owner of Dogma Grooming Salon & Spa,
and professional photographer

A heartbreaking story, written with great care. Fellow sufferers of IBD diseases will find in it both inspiration and healing.

—**Harriet Levin,** author of *The Christmas Show* and
winner of the Barnard New Women Poets Prize

It was an absolute pleasure to read Annie's story, to learn about her and the influence she had on those around her just by living life to the fullest. It is a very inspiring book in which Annie practically jumps off the page and wraps me in a hug. I found myself wanting to have conversations through the pages with Annie—a sign of a well-written, well-organized story.

—**Laura Sarasqueta,** For the Love of Editing,
Gilbert, Arizona

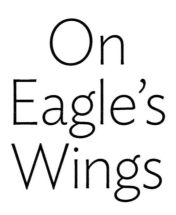

On Eagle's Wings

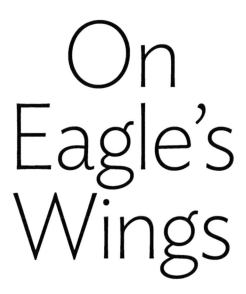

On Eagle's Wings

*The Inspirational
Life of Annie Stites,
Crohn's Survivor*

GAIL PARKER

From the life and journals of Annie Stites

In loving memory of
Annie Stites

Annie, you showed me in so many ways how to enjoy and appreciate life and that every day is a gift. You taught me that laughing over the worst calamities is better than crying over them and that those terrible calamities can make the best stories. And you made me even more aware that there is nothing in this world that is more important than love.

But those who wait on the Lord
Shall renew their strength;
They shall mount up with wings like eagles,
They shall run and not be weary,
They shall walk and not faint.

Isaiah 40:31

Contents

CHAPTER ONE

Leave a Footprint

"I want my life to count for something.
I want to leave a footprint that the tides of
time may fade but never fully wash away."
—ANNIE

MY NAME IS GAIL PARKER. Annie Stites was my sister—well, technically, she was my sister-in-law but we dropped the "in-law" soon after we got to know each other. I knew Annie from the time she was thirteen until she was sixty. Annie was the most exceptional person I have ever met. I have never been able to talk about Annie in only a few words, and in this book I don't intend to try!

There were so many parts of her life, it was as if she were many different people and each part of her life could have been its own story. Her lifelong romance with her husband, Glenn—also known by the nicknames "Hippie," "Lovie," or "Captain" depending on Annie's mood or the present situation—would be story enough, living as they did in a log cabin in the woods of Cape May Court House, New Jersey. Add to that her care for animals both domestic and wild, her sailing adventures, the charity she founded, her passion for working with special needs children and sufferers of the same Inflammatory Bowel Disease (IBD) that rocked her world so frequently, and you have a personality almost too big to be captured on the page.

Many people told Annie that she should write a book because her life was so extraordinary. Annie and I frequently talked about her writing a book while she was alive, but it never materialized for one simple reason: the double-sided coin of health and disease. When Annie was ill, she was too weak to attempt such a daunting project, and when she was well, she was too busy making up for lost time and living the very life that was worthy of a great book. When Annie was nearing the end of her life, I was possessed by the passion to write about her so that her life didn't end with death. Little did I know I would get some help from a very wonderful surprise . . . .

When Annie was in hospice care, I would frequently drive two hours each way from Philadelphia to be with her and then go on to the cabin where Glenn and I would sit poolside dangling our feet in the water, processing both our grief and our joy over Annie's remarkable life. I recorded many wonderful stories that he had to tell about their years together. After she passed away, we talked on the phone for many hours a day over the next several months; I would take notes during our conversations about Annie, and this proved helpful to the healing process for both of us.

One day when I was visiting Glenn, he told me that Annie had written many journals, and that I could take them home with me. What a surprise and a blessing! Annie had never talked about her journals and yet here were dozens of them—handwritten stories and her unique opinions all portrayed in vivid words. It was as if Annie's own voice had seemingly been brought back to life!

I took boxes and boxes of her life home with me and started a three-year journey of sifting through all of the thoughts, ideas, and stories that had flowed from Annie's mind onto the pages of her journals.

In Annie's words:

> *Years ago I started my journal for the sheer pleasure of writing. The challenge, the spark was ignited by my overwhelming enthusiasm and joy while cruising the Chesapeake aboard our beloved sailing vessel, Freyja [pronounced Freeya]. I was brimming over with almost childish glee, soaking up our surroundings. It was then I first felt the need to put these emotions on paper . . . .*
>
> *I can't remember a time when I wasn't intrigued with words, the symbols, the sounds, and the way one word could have different meanings.*
>
> *As a child, I enjoyed the illustrations of stories, but I was always more eager to understand and*

pronounce the words. It was the interplay that cre-
ated the images of the story that would pique my
interest and stir my imagination. It was the words
that created the pictures that truly illustrated the
story and brought the characters and settings to life.
And it was the combination of words that created
a brand-new experience.

How I perceived their denotation as well as
their connotation is what enabled each reading
time to provide the escape I so desperately sought
and needed given my home life, my recalcitrant
body, loneliness, confusion, and pain. Books
became my friends, and I enjoyed all types from
fiction to history.

Several times I came across Annie's belief that these
writings would never be read, even by her; she rarely
reread what she had written and certainly never believed
anyone else would read them. Annie questioned her
compulsion to write, saying:

Why write words that will never be read? If someone
talks out loud in an empty room, will their voice
be heard? If I fill a blank page with words and no
one reads them, do the words still have meaning,
truth, or value?

What is my motive for endlessly writing? Why
has writing become a compulsion? I am incomplete,
dissatisfied, and uncomfortable if I let too much
time pass without writing. Perhaps some of the

reasons are for venting or self-expression, or self-satisfaction or words that bring out the truth. The written word has veracity and validity. Writing it down somehow makes it true.

I enjoy the peaceful mechanics of writing, the simple movement of a pen across the page. Blank pages beckon me, encouraging me to fill them. I can talk on paper without consequences.

We both realized that writing a book would be too much of an undertaking for her to ever attempt on her own, and so we talked about writing the book together; she would tell me stories and I would do the rest but even that was too much for her near the end of her life. So after she passed, when I found out about Annie's journals filled with her stories and perceptions of life, it was then that I felt the synchronous hand of fate sweeping across both of our lives.

I have a question for me. Why, oh Lord, why do I always have this compulsion to write? I can never totally enjoy or truly experience a special time unless I write about it.

Oh, I yearn to write well, to express in words this life of mine, shaded and in the sun. I want to share the wonderful and not-so-wonderful chapters that make up the novel of my life. I write of daily things wanting to describe a walk through the meadow so well that the reader will be beside me. The book within me is pushing to be born.

As I selected the passages from Annie's journals for this book and worked on the narrative that would surround them, I knew that we had at last found a way to write the book of her incredible life together. I felt that I hadn't really lost Annie, that instead she would be forever with me, her family, her friends, and everyone who was going to read this book.

In one of her later journal entries, Annie wrote:

> *I desperately want my gift of life to be worthy of the miracle of my life. I am so humbled and grateful for you, dear Lord, allowing me to live. Here I am in my fifties, and I wasn't meant to survive my infancy.*
>
> *I want my life to count for something. I want to leave a footprint that the tides of time may fade but never fully wash away.*

The most remarkable thing about Annie was that her life did count for something, and something magnificent: she changed the life of everyone who was blessed to have known her. I have done the final piece of authoring this book in the hope that that circle of individuals would grow ever larger.

CHAPTER TWO
The Miracle Baby

HE FIRST TIME I MET ANNIE she was thirteen and sitting cross-legged in the middle of her bed, surrounded by an array of stuffed animals, schoolbooks, and papers. Clutched in her hand was the TV remote control.

The TV was her constant companion and staved off the great loneliness that was present without it. Annie had mastered the art of watching several shows at the same time, and old classic movies became her closest friends.

Her bed had become an all-too-familiar part of her life, and she sat on it like a queen ruling over her domain. Her blond hair was cut short and fell in one layer just past her chin. Her blue eyes were quite alive even though they were pink rimmed from lack of good health. Other than her blue eyes, Annie bore her father's features.

Annie tried to keep her journals positive and not give in to writing about the chronic disasters that were so often present among her family members. I would later come to know the whole story, and although Annie did vent on occasion, I personally witnessed how Annie's fascination with living always outweighed any bitterness she was experiencing.

I popped out of the womb attached to an IV. Born with a floating intestine that had a hole in it, I was literally about to die from the moment I was born. I had an intussusception where the large bowel was ingesting the small intestine. The doctor told my parents that he had to do an exploratory surgery, as it was my only hope and a very slim one at that.

My Gramma wrote to her cousin in December of 1948, "No one knows how this baby is hanging on. Every day appears to be her last; but then she pulls through. They resectioned part of her intestine, and her little veins collapsed under the strain. Poor little thing has many tubes running from her tiny legs and arms. We were ready to bury you, poor, tiny, sick thing. No, Annie, you were supposed to die, you were so ill . . . ."

The surgery was miraculously successful; in fact, I was dubbed the "miracle baby" at Jefferson Hospital in Philadelphia. My family had actually prepared a gravesite for me. I spent several months in the hospital before I was well enough to leave. When I was sent home after four months, it was because, as my parents were told, there was no more that could be done. I did not sit up until I was thirteen months old.

Several years went by, and my health stabilized and then improved. I thought of myself as just a normal kid, but my mother thought of me as a sickly child and was always, in my mind, needlessly cautious with me. I remember Mom screaming at my brother, Lowrey, who is seven years older than I am, as he was swinging me around by one arm and one leg out in the front yard. I was squealing with delight while Mom was yelling for him to put me down, saying that I was a sick child.

Her mother Jane's insistence on seeing Annie as impaired could not squelch Annie's spirit.

I had a close friend and we were inseparable. I have many memories of long, lazy Saturdays with Candy Worden holed up in her room with a week's allowance spent happily at Penn Valley Drugstore for penny candy, Sugar Daddy candies, and comics. Lulu, Archie, and Casper were rated favorites! Popcorn was at the ready for a salty munch between the sweets.

Of course if the day was just too nice to waste staying inside, we would be off to the woods, making fantastic forts. Closing my eyes now almost, gulp, thirty-five years later, I can still walk those familiar paths when I was pure in health between being deathly ill as a baby and when the first onset of Crohn's disease began at age twelve.

Dear Candy with shiny brown hair in a boyish bowl cut was forever propping her thick errant glasses back on her freckled nose because they were always slipping down as she tossed her head excitedly while telling me about a neat idea for a new project or adventure. Two large, slightly bucked front teeth were being corrected with braces, and she was always shooting off her rubber bands. Spit would go flying as she absentmindedly wiped her chin and put back the rubber bands. She would continue on with staccato sentences—the words couldn't come fast enough to explain her brainstorm.

We were soul mates, both tomboys who loved being outdoors, riding our bikes, whizzing up and down hills, rounding corners with legs outstretched, and gleefully yelling out raucous yahoos with our dogs barking at our heels, which at 8:00 on a Saturday morning rattled the suburban calm.

I can still remember the sheer, unfettered joy as I hopped out of bed on a Saturday morning with a whole day just waiting to be filled with new adventures. I would dress quickly, run downstairs two at a time, and dash off on my trusty Schwinn. Peddling fast, I could see the sidewalk rushing under me with strips of grass between the cracks, then thump, bump over the curb onto the empty, sun-dappled street leading to my friend's house.

Her home was always so warm and happy, full of teasing and laughter. I felt so safe there.

In contrast to the safety and happiness that Annie felt when she was at her friend's house, there was unrest at home, never knowing when fights would break out between her parents.

Alcohol became an increasing part of my parents' life. Their marriage became stormy and because both had strong personalities, their battles sometimes became physical. There were desperately sad times before Mom and Pops's divorce—the fights, the parties, the drinking, all very loud to this little kid and always frightening.

Our home at that time was an endless source of both large and small places where I could escape, giving vent to my boundless imagination.

I had little gnome friends. When a book of gnomes became popular years ago, I nearly jumped out of my socks. There, in exquisite detail, was a world that I had dreamed about as a child.

Perhaps there remains within each of us that special place within our souls, the carousel of brilliant, uninhibited child imaginings, those places and characters that were created so very long ago with such effortless ease. Natural springs would burst forth from our young minds, still unencumbered by adult webs of reality.

I used to sit under the huge willow in our back-yard amid the gnarled, knuckles of the roots. There among the moss and under the roots lived my little people with acorn shells, berry pits, and seedpods, all implemented for their houses. Even now, remembering makes me smile.

As a child, Annie called her father "daddy," which became "pops" as she grew older. This change most likely happened sometime after he left the house.

A defining day in my life was when I was eight years old and my father, whom I adored, stood with suitcase packed and told us he was leaving the house for good. I can still hear myself screaming, "Daddy, don't go, please, please don't go," as I was crying hysterically and pleading with him to stay. Lowrey, with tears in his eyes, had to pull me off of my father as somehow I thought if I could just hang on to him I could actually keep him from walking out of the door and out of our lives. Daddy finally broke away from my grip, and with my brother's arms holding me tightly, we watched as Daddy walked down the path to the driveway. After putting his suitcase in the trunk, he drove away without once looking back at us. I was devastated.

How blessed I was to have Lowrey as my brother. He had to assume a difficult role as father/brother when he was only a teen. Mom, my sister, Tyler, and I depended on him after Pops abandoned us, thinking only of himself and his needs. My childhood was happier because of you, Lowrey.

> *I still remember mischief night. Mom wouldn't let me out. I went to my room, slammed the door, and grabbed a doll as I prepared for a banner sulk. A few minutes later I heard a tap-tap on my window. I see my brother still, grinning his crooked smile, ears reddening with laughter and eyes with a mischievous twinkle. "Open up." He took my hand and pulled me onto the apex of the roof. I could still see in the pre-evening dusk. We scampered down the roof, jumped to the porch, and thumped onto the ground at a run. I felt so free! I ran down the side of the house, across the backyard, and climbed over the wooden gate, traversing backyards to get to my friends.*

It wasn't too long after that when I first met Annie. I remember going up to her bedroom and chatting with her for quite a while and finding her fun, warm, and friendly. There was no awkwardness even though we had never met before.

About a year after Annie's parents divorced, her mother, Jane, bought a smaller "twin" house, got a job, and started dating. Within a few years, Jane met Hughart Laughlin at an AA meeting. Hughart came from a lot of money. His family's business was Jones/Laughlin steel, and he grew up in Pittsburgh next door to the Melons. In spite of the fact that he was a graduate from Princeton University, his drinking kept him from having a prominent position in the family company. He was a salesman until he retired. Hughart never had to worry about a paycheck, however, because he had a trust fund that allowed him to live very comfortably.

When the decision was made to have Hughart move in with Jane, Annie was not asked if that would be all right with her. Annie was not at all happy about having another man usurping her territory. Jane gave all of her time and attention to Hughart, and Annie felt like a stranger in her own house. Many years later, after Hughart had passed, Annie had this to say about her relationship with Hughart:

> *There are barbs of bitterness and resentment concerning a total upheaval of my life, yet there was love and concern from Hughart later on. He was such a weak, pliable man and such a pawn for my mother, who was much too strong a personality for him. After the romance had died, she used to call him Mr. Melba Toast because he would walk away from a fight. I think Mom loved a good scrap and was used to it with my father. In order for her to respect a man, she needed him to stand up to her.*
>
> *Later I learned that Pops had been having an affair with my mom's best friend, Bobbie, who was also an alcoholic. The affair led to my father leaving my mother and us.*

After a quick divorce, Annie's father and Bobbie, who became "Aunt Bobbie" to his children, married and moved into a large old farmhouse. It sat on thirty-three acres and was referred to as "the Farm" It was also given the name Fivormor. The concept was that there were five of them: Annie's father, Bobbie, and Bobbie's three children. The "ormor" was allowing for another child—Philip, Jr.

In the summer, the pool was the center of their activities. In addition to dogs and cats, they owned two horses that grazed picturesquely in the pasture surrounded by a white rail fence.

The setting looked appealing, but as is often typical in second marriages, the mother's children are protected and favored by her, and the husband's children from a first wife become a threat.

During Annie's senior year in high school, the atmosphere in Annie's home had become hostile. Hughart was not used to living with a teenager and had unrealistic expectations, while Annie was rebellious, which caused fights between her and her mother. Jane feared for the safety of her relationship with Hughart and resented the threat that Annie posed. The day of Annie's graduation, she and her mother had a big fight. Her mother didn't show up at her graduation, but Annie's father was there. When Annie came home from the ceremony, she found that her mother had "gone off the wagon"—she was drunk and had thrown all of Annie's belongings out of the second-story window of Annie's room. The doors had also been locked, leaving a clear message that her mother didn't want her living there anymore. Annie was left with little choice but to go to her father's house, and it wasn't just for that night. Annie went to live with her father.

Moving to "the Farm" didn't eliminate Annie's home problems; it just relocated them. Annie never felt that she belonged at the Farm, and she was unhappy.

> *I always felt I was such an outsider, trying to please Aunt Bobbie with a nervous lump in my chest. Such lonely nights at the Farm. My bedroom was in the back wing and I thought of it as my sanctuary and my cell. There are still so many stark memories of walking through to my bedroom. Almost daily, Aunt Bobbie had a little gift for her children on their beds. I would go through to my room expectantly and found nothing. Oh, it wasn't the lack of getting a gift that upset me; it was the pang of knowing I didn't belong and never would. I would cover up my hurt with banter while shaking inside. Never could I tell Pops of these slights; it would just cause a fight.*
>
> *I was always nervous as I entered the drive— my heart pounding, loneliness and alienation never to be forgotten. As I would come up the steps from the driveway entrance, Aunt Bobbie would be seated at the kitchen table, chin resting in her hand with the ubiquitous cigarette swirling pearl gray smoke around her head. I would peek cautiously around the door into the yellow glow of the kitchen. Was I in trouble? Was I late? Had I forgotten something?*

When Annie was fifteen, I married her brother, Lowrey, and we had David and Lynnie—Annie's first nephew and niece. Thirteen years later Lowrey and I divorced and we both remarried. Lowrey married a woman with two children, Kari and Johnny. These children also became Annie's niece and nephew. After seven years that marriage dissolved, and Lowrey remarried a woman who had a daughter, Tori, and a son, Phil, adding another niece and nephew to Annie's family. Annie's sister, Tyler, had two children, AmyJane and Christian, and there were more nieces and nephews to come from Annie's half- and step-siblings.

I remained very close with Annie, and when I remarried, my very loving husband, Ray, and Annie developed their own special relationship.

A strange note about this large, dysfunctional family is that despite everything, they are a family with humor, love, and support for each other. And perhaps even stranger, my husband and I are still included in many parties that are hosted by Lowrey's side of the family, and we are friends with Lowrey and his third wife, Susie, which makes our own family celebrations enjoyable. It is always fun to shock strangers by revealing the unusual dynamics of our family when we are all together.

But when Annie was growing up, happy family celebrations didn't happen. In one of her journals, she talked about her childhood birthdays.

I enjoyed a peaceful, wonderful birthday yesterday.
For some reason my birthday has always made me

subdued and a bit depressed. Oh, not from the age bit—hell, I'm thrilled and grateful to have made it through one more year!

Mom never did much on my birthday. I never had a birthday party until I was sixteen. That was a memorable day with the Carlin family in Margate, New Jersey. They gave me my first party.

Annie's sixteenth year was also the year when Annie first began working with geriatrics as an aide at the Broomall Nursing Home. Annie worked there for two summers, and she loved it. Her ambition to become a nurse, however, was undermined by Crohn's. Although she was accepted at Jefferson School of Nursing, her doctor restored some passages in her health record that she had "forgotten" to put on her application.

I still remember the talk in his office. "Annie, dar-lin', you just couldn't make it through the rigorous study/work schedule. You would flunk out in a year." God, I was so totally crushed. I had wanted to be a nurse since I was twelve and reading the Cherry Ames nurse series. I always gobbled up any book that had to do with medicine.

The caretaker in me was not to be ignored, so I opted for teaching. Originally, I was advised that I would not be able to attend college because of my health. Two schools rejected me saying that I would be "wasting a seat." Being told "no" just doubled my determination. I went to Marjory Webster Junior

College in Washington, D.C., and from there went on to study at Ithaca College in Ithaca, New York, where I majored in English.

Flare-ups of illness throughout college required frequent hospitalizations. Colitis was diagnosed and treated with massive steroids and a strict diet. Would you believe that for two years I lived on rice and baby food? Liquid diet was no problem, however. Beer is a clear liquid, isn't it?

It took five years to finish college but I graduated! After my last final, I threw my books in the air and perforated right there on the quad. That action resulted in my first major Crohn's surgery. I received my diploma in 1971 in my hospital bed. The dean presented my diploma dressed in full cap and gown while my friends hummed "Pomp and Circumstance" from the hallway.

As soon as I could be transferred, which was two months later, I was taken to a Pennsylvania hospital in a hearse from Ithaca because there were no ambulances available. I entertained myself by occasionally putting my hand up to the window to wave at people in cars driving by just to freak them out.

I weighed eighty pounds and had multiple fistulas and peritonitis. I was operated on a second time and had a nightmare month in ICU, followed by another two months in the hospital.

After fully recovering I was able to get my own apartment and taught remedial reading for six months. I wanted to further my education, so I entered graduate school pursuing a master's degree by day and a Ph.D. at night in Special Education at Millersville College in Pennsylvania.

Again I had frequent bouts of pain, fever, and constant diarrhea. While lying on the living room floor typing the final copy of my thesis, I had a fistula and my stomach literally opened up and fecal matter shot out like old faithful. My brother raced from Philadelphia to come pick me up, and while enduring unbelievable pain, I finished my thesis and called my professor asking if he could come get it.

While Lowrey was breaking all speed limits getting me back to Philadelphia, in spite of my agony, I had to laugh when Lowrey showed his disgust at my cat when she crapped on his shoulder during the ride! The hospital had been alerted, and an OR was ready and waiting for me when we arrived. I had emergency surgery where they did a resection where the diseased part of the bowel is removed and healthy bowel is sewed together. It seemed that surgeries came in painful pairs. I could not heal properly at the site of the resection. Three more months were spent in the hospital.

My master's degree was unceremoniously sent to my home, and I came so close but never was able to complete my Ph.D.

Annie always had plans for the future, even if the future often had other plans for her. For example, Annie had a passionate desire to use her graduate degree to help children who had special needs. At first Annie took a job as a substitute teacher for one or two days a week. Then when a teacher quit, Annie moved into a full-time position working with mentally disabled children. Annie was there for about a year when the physical demands of working full time impaired her health to the point where she obstructed and landed back in the hospital with surgery.

After a couple of months in the hospital and several more months of recovery, Annie was again applying for a working position. She tutored students in math—something that made Glenn laugh because math had never been Annie's best subject.

Annie's tutoring job lasted for two years before she encountered more health problems. More surgery was necessary, followed by months in the hospital and then weeks of recuperation at home.

It was hard on Annie not to work. When she was well again, she went back to work as a substitute teacher and again, it turned into a full-time job and again, she obstructed and had surgery.

Sometime later, when health gradually returned, Annie began tutoring pregnant teenagers in their homes when they were no longer allowed to remain in school. The last time Annie took a full-time job, it was for Ocean Academy, working with profoundly mentally disabled children, many of whom were physically handicapped. She was accidentally kicked in the stomach by a boy who didn't have control of his muscles. Annie immediately doubled over with extreme pain, and the next day was taken to the hospital where she had extensive surgery.

She was never able to work for a school again, but she did eventually find her true vocation: counseling many people with ostomies and those facing IBD-related surgery. [An ostomy is the opening of the intestine through the skin of the abdomen with a bag attached.] The medical supply store would give her a call if someone was having a rough time, and she would go to their home or the hospital and talk with them. There wasn't an ostomy therapist in the local hospital, so when Annie made visits she would take catalogues and pull up her shirt.

> I have received a lot of phone calls from people who are suffering a lot from IBD and having real problems adjusting to it, going through guilt, denial, acceptance, the whole gamut. I have ten people ready to go in a new Crohn's support group.
>
> When counseling people on ostomies, I try not to use the old clichés of "you can do it." I try to be very honest with them about the effects of the surgery. It can be devastating, but only if you let it. You're not in control of your physical body, but you can make a choice. You can accept the surgery as a second chance at living and something that will improve the quality of your life. It's easy to become "me-centered." It's hard to see beyond the pain, the constant food-diarrhea chain. The surgery will enable them to look to tomorrow with hope. I ask them about their interests and what they like to do and encourage them by telling them that they will still be able to continue. I'm honest with others

about the disease so they're not dealing with any misconceptions. Other people take their cue from the patient. What I want them to understand is that whatever the limits they set on themselves, they're still in control of their life. They might have to modify their goals a little, but not completely. How you deal with this disease or this surgery is a matter of choice. You can choose to be depressed and defeated, or you can pick up your head and look around you to all the support of your family and friends and hang on to that love like a lifeline—for indeed, it is. I don't try to be a total Pollyanna. I know how difficult and frustrating this disease is and it can take over your life with fear and pain, but I try to show others by example.

I show ostomy patients pictures of me in a bathing suit or a slinky evening dress. You can wear anything you want. I never did look good in a bikini so that was no great loss there.

I've learned patience and endurance. I've learned how very precious time is. There is definitely a time to cry and a time to grieve when you're in pain, but there's also a time to laugh and a time to count your blessings.

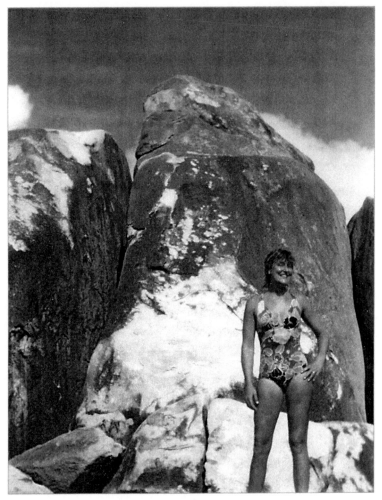

Would you believe this girl has an ostomy?

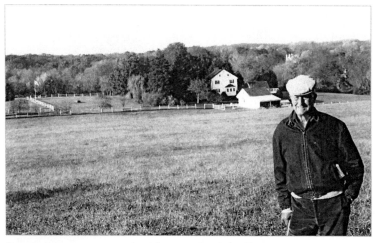

Pops in later years surveying his property at the Farm

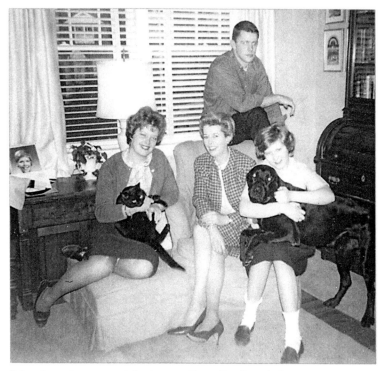

Tyler, Jane, Lowrey, and Annie sometime after Pops left

CHAPTER THREE

A Man of His Own Making

✤

WHEN ANNIE ATTENDED Ithaca College, she was briefly engaged. That prospective marriage ended when Annie was hospitalized with her first surgery for Crohn's disease. The boy's father was a doctor and advised his son that Annie was going to be sick for much of her life and it wouldn't be a good life for him. In retrospect, it is amazing to think that one surgery would scare someone off, but perhaps this was for the best; Annie would have twenty-eight surgeries in all and needed someone of the strongest character who wouldn't let her illness dictate how much time they would spend together.

Glenn loved Annie and that love meant that her illness was just part of who she was. He was willing to be there for her and with her through whatever future they would face together. They had far from a normal life, but although there were exceptionally bad times, there were also many exceptionally good times. God just may have had something to do with bringing Glenn into Annie's life.

The story of how this unique couple met is a romantic tale, made even more romantic because of the reality with which they had to contend. There is a large population from the suburbs of Philadelphia that spends as much time at the Jersey shore in the summer as possible. Family vacations are commonly enjoyed on the spacious beaches. Cottages are rented by the week, month, or season, and the wife and children live at the shore while the husband/father commutes on the weekends.

Living and working at the shore for the summer is almost a rite of passage for teenagers into their young adult years. There is something about the whole "shore" atmosphere that is addicting. After college, Annie found herself working in Avalon, an upscale shore town for the summer. She was staying with a friend whose parents owned a summer home there and started dating a friend of her friend's boyfriend.

One day when we were all together, the boys started talking about this guy they knew who grew up in Cape May Court House, a neighboring town. Apparently he lived in this incredible log cabin that he had built single-handedly. He was a carpenter, but he also had a little side business making unique sand candles. The boys had been to a couple of parties at his cabin and described them as great because he had several acres of property, creating a secluded setting. They called him a "longhaired hippie"—he always had some pot if you wanted it.

The boys thought it would be fun to introduce me to him and maybe wrangle an invitation to a party at his place, so we hopped in the car and headed for Cape May Court House. We turned down Highs Beach Road and started looking for the elusive dirt driveway that led to the cabin. When we finally found it, we parked outside the fenced-in yard, and as we came through the gate, we were greeted by Elka, the hippie's dog.

As we walked up the brick path, I remember being impressed and charmed by the rustic, two-story log cabin. Could one man really have built this all by himself? He had even dug out a large pond behind the house and had a slatted wooden patio in front of it.

We found their friend around back, busy making his sand candles. There were several boxes filled with sand that had negative impressions carved into them. To make the candles, wax of different colors was poured into the cavities and then wicks were set in place. He said he had learned this craft from a gypsy. There was quite a variety of styles, including a large hanging candle that had four wicks.

I was captivated with the whole ambiance of the cabin setting and this intriguing man. I found myself implausibly attracted to him at first sight.

He looked like someone out of a romance novel, and in my protected life I had never met anyone like him. He was six-foot-two to my five-foot-four. He had long wavy red hair that fell a few inches past his shoulders. His face was framed by a beard and mustache. Barefooted, he wore tattered blue jeans that sat low on his hips, and his shirtless body was tanned and well defined. I was also attracted to his carefree lifestyle and that he was a man of his own making.

Ironically, it was my boyfriend who introduced us.

"Annie, this is Glenn Stites."

Glenn barely looked up from his work to say hello. I stammered back a weak, "Hello," feeling my face flush.

We only stayed a few minutes but left with an invitation to join Glenn and a group of friends that were coming over to Glenn's cabin later in the week. When the four of us arrived at that party, we could hear music playing as we came up the brick walk. Several people were sitting around an outdoor fire pit having a good time, laughing, talking, eating, and smoking pot. The four of us joined in, and I found myself sneaking looks at Glenn throughout the evening. I observed that he was very relaxed and had a slow manner and delivery when he talked. He often paused for a few seconds with an "ahhh . . ." before speaking, as if he were carefully choosing his words. He was very laid back but laughed easily and had a subtle but good sense of humor.

> *I couldn't explain why, but just looking at him gave me butterflies.*

Whenever Annie told me about her first meetings with Glenn, I was always struck by her character: she was tenacious and not willing to give in or give up when there was something that she wanted, like her education or this particular man. She would somehow find a way to get it.

Glenn may not have been as prepared! Glenn is a Cape May County boy, born and raised. His family owned and lived in a six-unit apartment building where other members of his parents' family also lived.

Glenn's dad was a shipwright during World War II and built PT boats for the navy. Made from two layers of plywood that were glued and sewn together, they were considered disposable. The only thing that helped save these frail boats from total destruction was their speed. They had four engines and could go up to seventy miles an hour, which made them a hard target to hit.

Locked into his job, Glen's dad was never drafted because the war effort needed PT boats and men to make them. He taught Glenn all of his carpentry skills from an early age. In fact, the very first toy that Glenn remembers getting was a block of wood, a hammer, and a bag of nails.

In his family's apartment, Glenn had a large twenty-by-twenty foot bedroom on the third floor with its own outside entrance. When he was in eighth grade, he sectioned off part of the room and built himself a bathroom. His parents didn't want him to go to college, despite Glenn's IQ of 143. His father had plans for Glenn to work with him, and so he became a carpenter and later on a contractor.

In the late 1960s, Glenn was twenty-four and still living in his parents' apartment building and working with his dad. One morning a girl was seen leaving his room from the outside stairway, and he was told that he was not to entertain overnight guests in their house. That was the catalyst for Glenn to start looking for his own place to live.

He didn't have the money to buy a house, so he bought four acres of property set back in the woods in Cape May Court House and started building a log cabin. He designed the cabin and driveway around existing trees so as few as possible would need to be cleared. Used telephone poles were bought for seven dollars each, recycled one-inch steel crane cables were immersed in concrete for his footings, and New Jersey white cedar clapboard from a 120-year-old funeral home became the gable ends. After removing the nails, Glenn reversed the boards, turning the painted side against the cabin. The recycled windows were not the usual one-sixteenth-inch, but quarter-inch plate glass, which provided better insulation from the heat and cold. The floors were made of brick and concrete. Many of the materials used were leftovers from his construction jobs.

Glenn constructed the entire cabin single-handedly, including the electricity and plumbing. He only hired professional help to drill the well, set up the septic system, and install the furnace for the hot air heating system once he had completed all of the duct and masonry work.

To build a two-story log cabin by himself, Glenn had to be resourceful and innovative. Sixty-seven logs were dumped at the edge of his property. Glenn put together two car tires with a short axle between them. After lifting the small end of a log and chaining it to the axle, he could then roll a 12,000-pound log down the driveway. To hoist the logs into place for the cabin walls, he used surrounding trees with cables and pulley systems. Working at night and on weekends, it took about a year and a half to build the cabin.

> *Brought up on the Main Line of Philadelphia, where the well-schooled, wealthier people lived, Glenn was the antithesis of every boy that I had ever known or dated. Perhaps that was part of the attraction; I don't know. What I do know is that I took every opportunity to go back to that cabin throughout the summer!*
>
> *By the end of the summer, I had stopped seeing my boyfriend and had returned home to start working at Elwin Institute, a home for special needs children.*
>
> *My friend had become engaged, and she and her fiancé were temporarily living with Glenn at the cabin. I started going down to the cabin on weekends under the pretense of visiting my friend, but I had an ulterior motive.*
>
> *There was just one glitch: Glenn had a girlfriend.*
>
> *I continued to come down every weekend anyway. Returning home from his dates, Glenn would*

find me asleep on his couch. I remember he always made sure that I was covered before going upstairs to bed.

Several weekends went by and Glenn came to the end of the road with the girl he had been seeing. After their last date, they said good-bye and Glenn came home to find me awake. This was the first time that we had had any length of time together just the two of us. We sat and talked for quite a while. I admitted that I was glad that Glenn was not going to be seeing that girl anymore because I had been falling in love with him since the first time we met; he admitted that I was the reason that he had broken up with the girl he had been dating.

Giving in to all of the feelings that had been developing for the last several months, I pulled his face down to mine and kissed him. He kissed me back, and after a few minutes of building passion, I took his hand and led the way upstairs.

As my clothes came off, Glenn could see long scars on my stomach from previous surgeries. He noticed, but they didn't bother him. They were just scars. We made love with tenderness and passion. I could hardly believe what was happening. After months of wanting him, and Glenn being so different than any boyfriend that I had ever had or was expected to have, here I was in his bed, in his arms, and we were making love. The next morning we fixed breakfast together, and throughout the day we would look at each other and break into a grin.

By the end of the day, I had to drive back to Philadelphia for the workweek. I shared Glenn's bed every weekend for the next several months as our relationship grew. At last it seemed that everything was coming together in my life, and I was happier than I had ever been.

Because Annie was working at this time, she had an income and was able to get her own apartment with her stepsister, Peyton. Annie was at last teaching mentally challenged children. This was her passion and the culmination of all her daunting health struggles to achieve her education. The workweek was tiring but fulfilling. Annie and Glenn talked on the phone during the week, and Annie looked forward to Friday nights when she would drive the two hours to the shore to spend the weekend with Glenn. By this time, Annie's friend and her fiancé had moved out of the cabin to a place of their own. The weekends were relaxing and fun with no stress, which was just what she needed. After Annie would leave on a Sunday night, Glenn would be alone in the cabin for the rest of the week with just his dog, Elka.

Back when Glenn was still living in his parents' apartment house, he answered an ad in the paper for a purebred Norwegian Elkhound that was for sale. He had always wanted to have his own dog, and so he went to see her and found that the owners had been keeping her in the garage on a concrete floor. She was a year old, and her muscles were so weak from lack of any exercise that she couldn't go up stairs. Glenn bought her and took her home. He had to carry her up and down the two flights of stairs to his room until she gradually developed enough muscles to make it on her own. Glenn's grandmother, who lived in one of his parents' apartments, helped by walking Elka for increasingly longer amounts of time every day.

Glenn's grandmother was quite a person. Retirement was mandatory at age sixty-five at her job as a teller and secretary in a bank, but because she had falsified her age from the beginning, she continued to work until she was seventy-eight, at which time her little deception was discovered. As Elka gained normal strength, people would call to report that Gram and Elka had just been sighted passing their house, which could have been as far from home as four to five miles.

Elka was always with Glenn when he was working on the cabin, and when she rode in his old red pickup truck, she would sit in the middle of the bench seat, leaning against him.

Glenn furnished his new home with a few pieces of his grandmother's antique furniture and many pieces that he crafted from locust trees. Glenn never used screws in making his furniture; they were all put together with dowels.

A secondhand Franklin stove was given to him. At the time Glenn was grateful for the inexpensive heat. He had a lot of wood surrounding the cabin that he could burn.

Incredibly, just two months after Glenn and Elka moved in, a fire broke out and the inside of the entire cabin was gutted. Firemen arrived and positioned themselves to the side of each window, awaiting the signal that the water had been turned on. When the signal came, the firemen broke through the windows with their axes. All of a sudden an explosion of glass shot out from every window. The quarter-inch glass had provided an almost airtight condition that allowed the fire to feed only off of the oxygen that was inside the cabin—a very fortunate coincidence that contained the fire almost entirely to the inside. Spears of glass three inches wide at the top and pointed at the other end were later found embedded in trees up to fifteen feet away.

The firemen were puzzled as to how the fire could have gotten started given the safety protection that had been provided. A perfect V-shape burn on the outer log wall illustrated and confirmed that the source of the fire had come from the Franklin stove when its walls dangerously overheated.

Glenn later learned that the house where the stove came from had also burned down. He all too gladly took a sledgehammer to the stove and removed it from the cabin in pieces, making sure that it would never cause that kind of devastation again.

Glenn's disposition always has adapted well to adversity. He takes things in stride with an "it is what it is" attitude that would later serve him well during Annie's tumultuous health difficulties. So he just went to work getting rid of all the wet and burned contents in the cabin and then started repairing the log walls.

The charred surfaces of the logs had to be ground down with an angle grinder equipped with a stiff wire brush. The removing of the wet, charred wood made an overwhelming mess. Luckily the brick and cement floors were impervious to the heat and not damaged. Some rafters had been charred one-eighth-inch deep. After the charred wood was removed, they were sistered to another rafter for stability. After finishing all of the restoration work, Glenn hired a company to eliminate the chemicals that create the smell of smoke.

A few months later, after a lot of hard work, Glenn and Elka resumed their lives in the restored cabin. In retrospect, Glenn's childhood and the kind of person he would grow up to be, with his talents, disposition and ability to love deeply, led to the person who would become Annie's rock. This is Annie's story, but Glenn was such a big part of it. She never could have had the life she had without his love, acceptance of her health, skills to be able to work while still being there for her, and their common interests.

One morning in February 1975, I was on my way to work when a car breaking the speed limit blew a stop sign—the horrible accident that ensued resulted in the gearshift being lodged in my intestines. Crohn's went bonkers! The emergency surgery for total obstruction was unsuccessful and I almost died. There was no choice but for an ileostomy to be performed, and I was hospitalized for the next five months.

This was not only physically traumatic, but also emotionally devastating when you are newly in love and now suddenly disfigured for life. It was a perfect scenario for a legitimate lawsuit, but Pops said that no child of his was going to sue anyone and he wouldn't allow it. At the time he said that he would take care of my financial needs, but those turned out to be only words. Was he sparing the insurance company or his reputation? My life would have been so much easier with financial backing to help with the future loss of work and hardships that were to come.

While I was in the hospital for five months, Glenn made the trip to Philadelphia as often as possible to be with me. Still recuperating and extremely weak, I was discharged and went home to the apartment I had been sharing with my stepsister. Peyton was young, working, and not prepared to be a caretaker. She knew how much I loved animals and without thinking of the possible consequences gave me the homecoming present of a baby raccoon we named Maude. I couldn't even properly care for myself, let alone take care of a wild baby raccoon!

During the time that I was in the hospital, my stepmother, Bobbie, had removed money from my bank account to pay for my portion of the rent. Now I had very little money left to live on. I hadn't worked for five months and was not going to be able to go back to my job anytime soon, if ever. My savings was running out. When necessary I would go out for just a few groceries, as I couldn't carry much, and would come back exhausted. As a last resort, I drove forty-five minutes to apply for food stamps.

That was the proverbial straw that caused Glenn to call.

"Annie," he said, "pack up a few things, I'm coming to get you. You can't stay there with no one to take care of you."

Glenn got in his old, red pickup and headed for Philadelphia with Elka at his side. When he got there he loaded me, a few of my belongings, and Maude into his truck and brought us back to the cabin to give me the care that I needed. Glenn really was the knight in shining armor and his steed was that old red pickup truck . . . .

That night Glenn tenderly took me to bed and made love to me. I was self-conscious about revealing my body and felt certain that the ostomy bag would be a turn off. I had prepared as best I could by folding the bag over and carefully placing a cinch belt over it that was five to six inches wide.

As we began to make love, the belt fastener kept pinching Glenn's stomach and he said to me, "Annie, let's get rid of this silly thing. I don't care if you shit out of your armpits, I love you."

That was the last time I ever tried to cover my ostomy, and I began my road of being able to provide hope and confidence to other ostomy patients.

Annie and Glenn lived happily together with their growing menagerie of animals at the cabin; Annie had fallen deeply in love with her backwoods hippie. Glenn was gentle, kind, and loving and took excellent care of Annie. The laid-back life at the cabin was perfect for her health.

One day, while doing some errands, Glenn said, "Let's go over to that jewelry store across the street and see what we can find."

They became engaged and planned a winter wedding when jobs were slow, giving them plenty of time to plan the ceremony and enjoy a ten-day honeymoon in Jamaica.

The date was set for January 17, 1976. They were married at Calvary Baptist Church in Ocean View, New Jersey, which had been Glenn's family church. I was honored to be one of Annie's bridesmaids, just as Annie had been in my wedding. At the Gold Club, where the reception was held for 100 guests, they were not allowed to have an open bar. It was, however, permissible to have a champagne toast. Glenn then brought in enough champagne for every guest to toast with his or her own bottle. That was typical of Glenn—a man who could usually find a way to work around a dilemma.

Despite having grown up in a suburban environment, Annie was well suited for cabin life. Born with a love for animals and nature, she had learned a lot from reading, so it was easy for her to wholeheartedly embrace Glenn's way of living, and make it her own.

I just came back from a happy discovery time with my neighbor's two children. We went owling in the backwoods. I threw Jimmy and Ryan off their couch and off we went for an adventure. We spotted two hawk nests, which sent Ryan and Jimmy scurrying with eyes downward in search of signpost "whitewash" or, in the vernacular, owl poop.

There were shouts of glee. "Come over here— there's piles of the stuff!"

I gamely, though not gracefully, clambered through the thorny thickets toward the treasure, looking upward, scanning the green cone-laden boughs hoping to see the singular silhouette of an owl, while knowing the chances were slim to none because of the racket we were making.

"C'mon, Annie, quick, an owl's been here. I know it."

"Okay, guys, now keep looking. Owl pellets, remember, fur balls."

"Yuck, that's gross."

"No, Jimmy, it's neat, really. An owl will swallow their food whole and chuck up the indigestible bones and fur."

I finally managed to stumble over to them, arriving with a plop on the ground as my sneaker snagged on scrub holly. Sure enough, promising white splats encircled the mighty shaggy pine. The copious amount made my adrenaline pump.

"Guys, this fellow roosts here a lot. There must be pellets around. They regurgitate every six hours. Look farther out from the trunk under the branches. It will be a furry ball, or it might be spread out. There . . . there, don't step on it, Jimmy, go ahead and pick it up."

Ryan was scampering through the thicket with his blue sweatshirt catching on thorns, impatient and excitedly shouting, "I'm coming, Jimmy. I know there's pellets, I can feel it, right, Annie?"

"Yep, look all around and don't shout," I shouted.

Jimmy picked up the mysterious wet gunk of fur with a bemused grimace and gingerly put the find in Ryan's outstretched palms. Ryan immediately squished and sorted through the gray wet mass.

"Here, Annie, here, bones, a claw, a tooth; neat, what was it?"

"I dunno, could be a vole or a skunk. I know there is more, guys, keep looking."

With heads down we all set to work scanning the forest floor, brushing aside thick layers of brown pine needles and leaves. Ryan, having come up with evidence of a squirrel, proudly handed me an acorn shell.

Within minutes came an excited cry from Jimmy. "Annie, Ry, here is another fur ball."

Ryan, my budding naturalist, jumped forward, eagerly grabbing the new treasure.

"Wow! Jackpot!" Wet and round, large bones were protruding, exposing a long leg with a joint knuckle still attached.

My admonition was mingled with praise when I told them, "Promise to respect this area, Ryan and Jimmy. We are intruding on the owls' territory. Great Horns lay their eggs in January, and the beginning of March is when the babies hatch. A female may *be on her nest right now, crouched low so we can't see her. Please, please, guys, don't disturb her. The babies will die if she leaves and you can scare her so easily. We will get a scope."*

At one point I demonstrated radar ears: I told them that by cupping your hands behind your ears you can listen to the woods' sounds.

We happily stuffed our pockets with fur and bones. "Your mom is going to love me for this, guys. We'll bring a baggie next time."

Pleased with our findings and with pockets full of treasures from the woods, such as "coins" of the Realm Acorn, a mysterious beige chip glued to a pine needle, two down feathers, assorted bone fragments in fur wrappers, and a twig with paint splash "whitewash," we headed home.

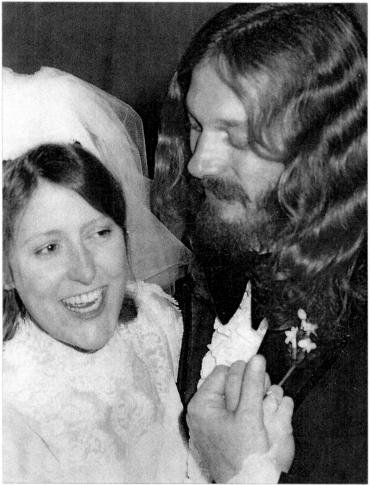

The happiest day of their lives

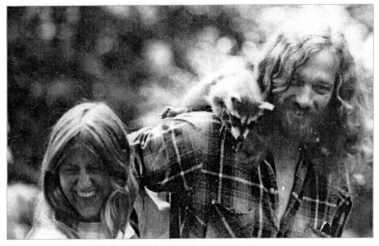

Annie being playful with Glenn and their raccoon

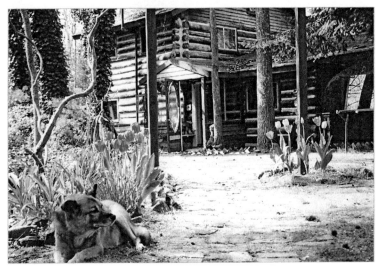

Spring at the cabin

CHAPTER FOUR

I'm Here to Have a Pedicure

WHEN SHE WAS FORTY, Annie was approached by the Philadelphia chapter of the National Foundation for Ileitis and Colitis. They were part of an organization that was sponsoring the "Great Comebacks Award™," and they believed Annie was a great candidate for the program as she had an unusually incredible story to share with others who were battling the same disease. A representative came to visit Annie in the hospital a few weeks after one of her many surgeries with an application in hand. Because Annie was still too weak to write at that time, she dictated her story into a microphone that Glenn held for her for a few minutes at a time over a period of several days.

They both got a kick out of the part of the application that asked for a "brief medical history." Annie began her answer to this question:

The phrase "brief medical history" certainly isn't analogous to Crohn's disease, but I'll try!

The first symptoms of Crohn's appeared when I was twelve with erythema nodosum, which presents itself as painful red lumps on my legs. My condition was first diagnosed as spider bites.

There were also arthritic symptoms of joint pain and swelling, like cigar fingers. I was given total bed rest (à la bedpan) and had a hospital bed in my room for ten months. I made it to school on the first and last day of seventh grade.

Throughout junior and senior high school, I had multiple bouts of Crohn's, still undiagnosed, missing three to four months of school a year. My senior year I was too weak to go a full day so I went half a day, taking major subjects in the morning, then home for a nap and back for after-school activities. All my friends were on sports teams. Not wanting to be left out, I became the team manager. I had homebound instruction because I refused to be held back, and in 1966, I graduated with my class.

Crohn's has never remained in remission for long in my life. My bowels will kink over on themselves causing total obstruction or a fistula. This always causes a King Kong–type pain. There have been frequent hospitalizations, two to four months at a time with IV feedings. Surgeries are performed, either resections or adhesion scrapes.

In between abdominal surgeries, I have managed to work in nerve replacement surgery on my arm, a total hysterectomy following my second miscarriage, and a proctectomy, a thirteen-hour surgery that left me hospitalized for five months. I have been on hyperalimentation multiple times and at one point was not able to eat anything solid for six months from August until February. I was sucking on the bed sheets! I have twice had a Candida infection, which is a fungus that enters the bloodstream from the catheter site of the hyperalimentation; this infection is life threatening, causing severe nausea and pain throughout your body.

I have had staph infections, during which my whole belly had to be opened up, and surgery for debridement of the wound was performed. The wound was left open, allowing it to heal from the inside out. It was very unpleasant emotionally as well as physically having my stomach laid open.

Another time a fistula that had formed next to my ostomy caused the need for yet another surgery. Experimental medication was tried to hopefully heal the bowel without operating. I spent two months on sump pumps, belly drains, and hyperalimentation. I could have been the centerfold for Popular Mechanics! The surgery that followed was to resect the bowel and reconstruct the ostomy. They were unable to save the ostomy, and I woke up with an unexpected new ostomy on the other side. I went

*to sleep with an ostomy on the starboard side and
woke up with one on the port side.
It was a long recovery but I made it!*

Annie had the marvelous ability to forget the bad times each and every time she emerged from a surgery, hospitalization, or complication. I never once saw her waste a moment of time when her health had returned (and by health, I speak relatively). She clung to feeling good with a fierce determination to enjoy life. After she relished a healthy period, her passion for living probably caused her to ignore each two- to three-month period in which—in reality—she was going downhill. She would stalwartly refuse to acknowledge or admit that a job, house, or whatever, was draining her body again and that an obstruction, Crohn's, was gearing up for its opening night, which would usually burst on to the scene during a January or February blizzard.

When an obstruction did occur, Glenn would take Annie to have a quick "shot" stop (for pain medication) at the office of her primary care physician, Dr. Haflen, who would come out to the car to give Annie a shot to help with the agony of the two-hour ride to Philadelphia. Then Glenn would drive them like a mad man to HUP, the Hospital of the University of Pennsylvania, while Annie was throwing up, rolling in agony, but still insisting on a self-destructive demolishing of a burger and fries! She knew that food would be the first thing taken from her and that there would be many days—sometimes months—with no eating. This routine changed little over the course of

Annie's adult life, altered only by variations among the
type of surgeries she endured or the length of the period
of time during which she felt relatively healthy.

*There is a burst of pain followed by tears of fear
and frustration. Oh God, what is happening to
me? Pain pills definitely help. It is okay if I sit here
and don't move. I really don't know what we are
going to do this time. I just can't do this to Glenn.
He needs all his time at work. I'm not going to think
of possible hospitalization—yes, the pain is that
bad. This is just not the time for this crap. I don't
think I am obstructing; the pain is too sharp for
that. It seems to be related to movement. I'm going
to see how the day goes. Maybe it's just a flare-up
of adhesions. Crohn's is not active; I only have one
lump on my leg. Oh God, please let this pass, and
I will concentrate on positive energy flow—I will
unravel negative thoughts and toss them away . . . .*

    *Pain is pretty bad still. Pretzel position assumed
for the duration—a bit terrified of what the consequences of this bout with the bully will be. I've taken
pain meds twice already just so I can function. Shit,
I refuse to face it. I will go on as long as I can. Pain
is reminding me that time is short and uncertain.
I have prayed for trust and patience—I must work at
reclaiming and retaining each precious moment . . . .*

    *Finally one gray morning in the beginning of
November, I decided I had had enough pain. I called
knowing full well that they would have to admit*

me; thus, the HUP sleigh ride began. I was put on a gastro floor and checked and rechecked by a nervous gang of med students. Oh, the endless stream of questions, repeated answers that were misunderstood and reexplained. All while I was in considerable pain and ready to explode if one more dork with a clipboard and "new doctor" tag entered my room.

"Umm, says here you have Crohn's, diagnosed when?" he asked and I answered.

"All that surgery," he continues, "ummm, you've had your share, huh. So, why are you here?"

I almost say, "To have a pedicure."

"You look like you don't feel well."

I want to respond, "Really, I'm ready to party, just stepped off a Princess cruise."

"Let's have a look," he says as he masterfully uncurls the stethoscope ceremoniously wrapped around his neck and places it on my chest.

Gad, my thoughts continue, don't you get circulation to your hands?

"Breathe in . . . let it out." Now there are two ways to wear a stethoscope, looped over your neck, definitely the cooler way, or curled into a knot in your jacket pocket. Now comes the ticklish situation: Do I untie my gown or just let this inexperienced med student grope and get tangled in it?

Sometimes I feel like I am the first warm patient any of them has examined, somewhat different than the black-and-white sketches in their books!

At HUP, Annie was blessed to have been delivered into the care of Dr. John Rombeau, a world-recognized leader in his field, who joined the faculty at the Hospital of the University of Pennsylvania as its first board-certified colon and rectal surgeon in 1979 and was promoted to professor with tenure in 1994. His special interests were Inflammatory Bowel Disease (Crohn's disease and ulcerative colitis), colorectal cancer, and diseases of the colon and rectum.

Dr. Rombeau was responsible for saving Annie's life multiple times and became a friend as well as her surgeon. It was Dr. Rombeau who performed the proctectomy that Annie mentioned in her application for The Great Comebacks Award.

In Dr. Rombeau's own words, "Postoperative survival in patients undergoing major surgery for Crohn's disease is not as good as non-Crohn's patients and during a proctectomy. It was necessary to create an omental sling or apron using this normal fatty covering on top of the small intestine to prevent the small intestine from subsequently obstructing by twisting deeply in the pelvis in the absence of a colon and rectum."

The proctectomy and creating a sling was a thirteen-hour surgery. Dr. Rombeau explains by saying, "It is not unusual for complex operations for Crohn's disease to be very time-consuming. The reasons for this are multifactorial and relate to the anatomic location and severity of ongoing disease, the effects of previous operations, which often distort the normal anatomy and impair exposure, and the presence of comorbidities such as nutritional status, weight loss, etc."

He also modestly gives credit to his skill by saying, "I was very fortunate to have been taught by world experts in Crohn's surgery at the Cleveland Clinic (Rupert Turnbull and Victor Fazio). The techniques I learned from these great surgeons indirectly benefited Annie. I guess this is what medicine is all about."

And then Dr. Rombeau touched on one of the most important reasons that Annie continued to survive: her own courage and will to continue living even after multiple surgeries and horrendous pain. "The most important lesson I learned from Annie is the important role of the psyche on clinical outcome. Patients who are determined to get well simply do better. They get out of bed sooner, eat better, and 'push' themselves to survive. To my knowledge, this observation defies physiologic explanations. Regrettably, the converse of this behavior occurs as well with ensuing poorer outcomes."

Dr. Rombeau's care of Annie was so profound that it prompted Annie's father, Philip Heaver (Pops), to write him this letter:

Never in all of my experience have I known of a surgeon who has shown the true caring for his patient as you have given to Annie before and after the operation. Certainly you are a skilled surgeon, but there is a deep dimension in you that surpasses the mechanics of the operating theater. In the eyes and grateful heart of this father, you're more than a credit to your surgical profession. You are a giant among men because you additionally offer an abounding measure of compassion and understanding to those who suffer.

Throughout Annie's long stays in HUP, not only Dr. Rombeau but also other attending physicians, nurses, and orderlies grew to love her. Her courageous and upbeat spirit quickly won them over, and her humor made caring for her enjoyable.

Unfortunately, this level of care was not uniform among all of the medical professionals who treated Annie. One time Annie had to be talked out of signing herself out of a hospital because a nurse got offended when Annie used a strong curse word. Annie had been trying to explain that she has an unusually high tolerance for pain medication and that she needed more than the nurse was giving her. The nurse didn't understand her history and had no idea what she had been through, or her level of pain and tolerance for pain medication. She either wasn't giving her the right meds or wasn't giving her enough of them. She thought two Percocet would do and for Annie, that would be like giving her two aspirin. After several attempts to enlighten the nurse to no avail, and while she was suffering terrible pain and becoming increasingly frustrated and exasperated, Annie finally gave up in despair and said, "Oh fuck it." That caused the nurse to sharply reprimand Annie for her language. The nurse seemed to be more concerned with Annie's expletive than her pain; that was the last straw for Annie, and she declared that she was leaving the hospital if she had to sign herself out. Glenn had to talk her down because Medicare would not pay if she were to sign herself out.

Then there was the time when it was expedient to take Annie to a local hospital, and there she received the worst care of her medical career. She had to fight against nurses who were about to put her in jeopardy because they had not reviewed her medical history. (Over the years Annie had become extremely knowledgeable about her disease, her body, and her medications.) Glenn was not allowed to stay with her, so Annie had to be her own advocate. In a threatening situation like this, Annie literally had to fight for her life like a cornered animal and throw niceties and proper language out the window.

It was Saturday and a beautiful screaming blue-sky day. I had clambered up to our roof to bird-watch. I had just finished telling a worried Glenn, "I'm okay, babe." The next thing I know I lost my footing, fell backward through the window, and my ribcage got hung up on the windowsill. I felt and heard a sickening rip and snap. I actually saw stars.

Somehow I made it through that night and the next day because I refused to go to the ER at Burdette hospital on a Sunday. Monday morning, I woke up with agonizing bolts of pain, making it almost impossible to breathe. The pain was exactly like post-op pain, ripping and searing down my side. All I could do was scream each time I took a breath. Glenn called an ambulance, and I was taken in spite of my protests to our local, loosely termed, hospital.

What ensued was more like Keystone doctors. Gad, what a mess. The nurse who admitted me was abrasive and unnecessarily rude. She made no eye contact and asked questions mechanically from an admittance sheet, pausing only to ask for spelling of the medications. I was in such pain and the smells, sounds, and the whole sterile environment triggered long-buried memories of past hospitalizations. Being apart from Glenn, and now to make it worse, spring was coming. Oh God, not now!

The nurse was talking to the orderly in between questioning me. "Oh yes, I got an extra large T-shirt for the marathon."

Then turning to me, she asked, "Allergies?" And continuing her conversation, "No, it wasn't raining in D.C. I would have run anyway."

After being admitted, I was taken to a room and managed to get myself on a gurney. A few minutes later, a nurse came in. She never got my proper medical history as she apparently had not read my admittance forms, and I could only whisper in short gasps from searing pain. I thought I had a punctured lung.

"What? Speak up, Mrs. Stites, I can't understand you. Any allergies?" she asked as she turned on her sneaker and walked away. A few minutes later she came back with a syringe.

I gulped. "What is that?"

"Pain med," the nurse answered. "I know, but what dose? What is it?"

She pulled me over onto my broken rib side. I screamed "NO" as she pulled off the protective needle cap with her teeth, taking aim. "Vistaril," she answered.

"I can't have Vistaril given with narcotics as a potentiate," I screamed out through clenched teeth.

"You can't be allergic to Vistaril. "

I blindly reached behind me to push her arm away, which caused an agonizing stab of pain.

"Don't you touch me, Mrs. Stites," the nurse responded. "And stop screaming."

I was in the room with one other man; poor guy, he must have thought he'd been dropped into a bad B movie.

"What is this scar on your buttocks?

"Vistaril, I told you."

"What?" as she lifted the needle up.

"I get a bed sore and then lose the feeling forever in the area of the shot." I tried to describe the reaction I get, a dead open sore that has to be scraped and drained. I had lost feeling in my thigh permanently from the last injection I received at Presbyterian hospital.

"Well," she said with disdain and disbelief, "I've never heard of that."

"Glenn, Glenn, get my husband now!" I needed Glenn to protect me.

"No, no visitors are allowed back here; there's not enough room."

My mouth was so dry—cotton mouth— that I was barely able to swallow. "May I have a little water?"

"No, you can't have water."

"I won't swallow it, just rinse my mouth out and spit. Please, my mouth is too dry." I could not swallow, and my lip stuck to my teeth.

A sense of foreboding swept over me. I actually felt at risk for my life. I was having so much pain I could barely move or speak up. I panicked and told the nurse to get out.

"Quiet, you are not the only person here. There is no reason to be so uncooperative, Mrs. Stites."

Empowered by sheer terror and rage, I climbed over the bars, and with my dehumanizing hospital gown flapping in the wind, I shuffled down the long hall, you know, the surgical walk with the body in the shape of a question mark, head bowed toward toes and eyes focused upward in a Frankenstein gaze. Through a door I staggered with the damn thing nearly crushing me.

Then I spied my precious redhead in the ER waiting room. No sooner had I yelped "Glenn" than a hard cold hand forced me down with a thud into a wheelchair.

"Miss, you are not allowed here! You are not going to fall on my shift!"

"Get your hands off me, I just want my hus-band, he doesn't know what is going on. You don't

know what we have been through. Please, please.
He is right there." I pointed a shaking hand toward
the lobby. As soon as I saw Glenn, I started to cry
and each sob brought a fiery stab of agony.

"Get security, I have an unruly patient." I could
not believe my ears or eyes as two security guards
came down the corridor toward me.

This can't be happening. "Oh Glenn, please, I'm
losing control." Fear and panic had caused seizures
and as my chest heaved I felt excruciating pain.
With great relief, I felt Glenn's large warm hand
on my shoulder.

The nurse was furiously sputtering "I never . . .
no need." I looked up at her and a stone-cold, calm
voice came from deep within me and I said, "Get a
grip, lady, I'm a patient, not a criminal."

Something in my demeanor caused her to stop
midsentence, jaw open.

The whole experience, which continued with an unhelpful and inept doctor, was like a Hitchcock movie for Annie. She vowed to never return to this local hospital. Annie was grateful that at her "home" hospital, University of Pennsylvania, the staff seemed to be aware that simply kind treatment can make such a difference in a patient's hospital experience and that a positive attitude toward healing is so important. They understand how scared the average patient is. Patients are in an alien environment, in pain or very ill, and some of them are deeply afraid. What they need are simple actions like using a soft voice, making eye contact, using a patient's first name, and being encouraging and compassionate—this can make a huge difference. A hospital experience is dehumanizing enough. For patients who are hospitalized for long stays, months at a time, the nurses and doctors become almost like a family to them.

At HUP, just before any of her surgeries, they allowed Annie to wear her wedding necklace until just before the operation began. The necklace was a symbol of Annie and Glenn's love, their strength, and their commitment to each other. Because Annie was a frequent surgery patient, Glenn was permitted to walk holding Annie's hand beside the gurney, farther than was usually allowed. When he was permitted no farther, he would bend down, his eyes brimming with tears, and with trembling fingers, too big for the miniscule clasp, take off the necklace and show it to Annie.

"I'll put this back on as soon as you wake," Glenn would say.

The deep-seated fear, terror knowing I might die and leave him sweeps over me. Then I look into his worry- and love-worn face and I know that the Lord won't separate us. The sheer force and depth of his love mirrored in his handsome, character-lined face strengthens me. We pray together with the tear-choked words calming and reassuring us.

The Lord is my shepherd, I shall not want. He maketh me to lie down in green pastures. He leadeth me beside the still waters. He restoreth my soul. He leadeth me in the paths of righteousness for his name's sake. Yea, though I walk through the Valley of the Shadow of Death, I will fear no evil for thou art with me; thy rod and thy staff, they comfort me . . . . Surely goodness and mercy shall follow me all the days of my life and I will dwell in the house of the Lord forever.

Our emotions are deep and sometimes we fumble over a line or two of the comforting message but trust and hope calms and strengthens us. We both cry as I give his hand one last squeeze. He reaches down and kisses me, and I am wheeled off to the operating room.

Hours later a bolt of searing pain makes my eyes burst open. Vision is blurred by anesthetic and pain. I seek Glenn. I look for that strawberry blond wavy hair. A warm hand covers mine as that precious face bends over me. "I'm here, Annie; we made it through another one. You are okay." My next sensation is his gentle touch as he puts my necklace back on.

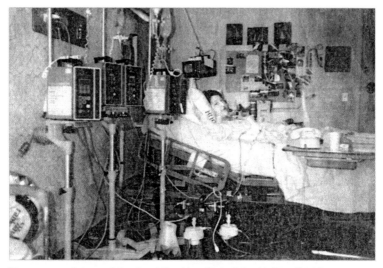

Newspaper picture of Annie at the Hospital of the University of
Pennsylvania, winter of '87, after twenty-three surgeries

CHAPTER FIVE

Snug in My Heart

❦

*T*HERE IS MORE OF COURSE that could be written about the double-sided coin of Annie's health and illness—in fact it could take up the entire book! And while her medical condition forms an essential backdrop to her story, of equal interest to my mind are the skills that Annie used to be able to cope with the difficult hand she had been dealt.

Why she didn't give up time after time I will never know! The only answer to that is that the intense joy of her good times outweighed the agony of the bad times. She was indeed a most exceptional person who used certain coping skills to focus more on the positive. One of the most enduring and effective of these was her faith.

The pain now is paralyzing me physically and psychologically after waking up to an explosion of smelly wet shit covering the bed and me. The smell alone was foul enough, and I could not move to help myself. Bolts of searing agony would make my body freeze.

I gritted my teeth, knowing there was no choice, and screamed involuntarily as I pushed off the filthy bed, getting shit all down my leg, and plopped into the wheelchair, fouling that up too, while still screaming.

I don't know where to put the excruciating agony. I walk to the toilet from the hallway because the chair won't fit through the doorway of the bathroom and am spreading a poop trail that I'm unable to clean up. I am also unable to get my pj's off—they are full of crap and wet and smelly! Such a wave of disgust and repulsion washes over me. I try to quiet my screaming child/woman within.

The appliance is now on the floor, staining the newly cleaned rug. Adding to my agony is the acid from the poop that is eating through my skin. The four-inch circle of raw, exposed, weeping, and bleeding, horribly painful skin around an almost flat stoma will not allow the adhesive disc on the appliance to adhere for more than a short period of time before breaking free.

Glenn had to cut my pj's off because I couldn't raise my arms or legs. I started singing hymns with the wrong words to an original melody I'm sure. Scripture always calms the pain.

Satan was scoring a field-long touchdown.
I want to die now. Too much, just too much! I can't
help but feel degraded when I can't care for myself.
I thought it was 7:30 p.m. but it was a.m., and poor
Hippie woke up yet again to a screaming me.
I am discouraged and afraid, and because of
the intensity of my agony, I worry about ruining
Glenn's life.
Enough of my venting, I am alive! I am grateful
to be thinking and writing again, and I will heal with
God's grace. Trusting Him, embracing His word,
praying, drawing on the Kingdom within the power,
courage, loving and being loved.

Perhaps faith is not actually a coping "skill," in the sense that Annie would have described her faith more as a gift that came from God to return her to her higher power, a source of strength and hope. But to me it can be described as a skill in part because it had to be nurtured and it had to start somewhere. The longer I knew Annie, the more I could see that her enduring faith came from her Gramma.

I had the delightful experience of first meeting Gramma, Frances Tyler Heaver, soon after Annie's brother, Lowrey, and I were married when we drove from the suburbs of Philadelphia to Gramma's home in Baltimore for a visit. I already had a loving picture of his Gramma from hearing him talk about her, and I couldn't wait to meet her.

In my childhood I had only known one grandparent. I was four years old when my grandmother came to live with us, and her mind had already pretty much slipped away. She died about a year later. I was told that I used to help her pull up her stockings in the morning and help her dress, but this—as with all other memories—is faded at best.

Gramma's home was warm and welcoming. There was a big, sprawling front porch where I was told she could be found on any given summer's day at 6:00 a.m., sitting in her rocking chair and reading from her Bible. Religion was very much a part of Gramma's life, and even well into her eighties she taught adult Sunday school in the Baptist church where she had been a founding member.

We pulled up to her large, white frame house with green shutters, and there she was, waiting on the spacious porch to greet us. I loved her at first sight. Frances Heaver was my picture of what a grandmother should look like: the stereotypical grandmother of yesteryear, a little taller than average height, full figured, wearing a comfortable dress, stockings, and sensible heels. Her thick wavy gray hair was neatly styled, and her face was properly wrinkled but cared for with a soft rosy blush and red lipstick. Gramma's blue eyes danced as she greeted me. As we hugged, a light scent of lilacs filled my senses. She welcomed us into her home with her old faithful dog at her side.

The ambiance of her house was warm, inviting, and old-fashioned, completing the essence of Gramma. Photographs were abundantly displayed, filling the house with memories of the family that she had raised there.

Many years earlier, after her husband had died, the large three-story house had been converted into a first-floor living space for Gramma's use, and the second floor was turned into an apartment that was rented for the purpose of having someone else living in the house to give Gramma a sense of security. The third floor was used for storage. We sat in her living room and chatted as I drank in the grandmotherly atmosphere of my surroundings. Lowrey loved to tease Gramma, and she would respond with a warm, gentle laugh saying, "Oh, Lowrey," in her soft Baltimore, Southern accent.

Grandma had prepared a lovely dinner for us, and I still have the recipe written in her own handwriting that she gave me for her delicious creamed mushrooms.

Driving back home, I realized how much I missed having a grandmother like Frances Heaver. Gramma lived to the ripe old age of 97 and after she passed, Annie wrote about her as she often did in her journals.

Gramma's love is the eternal treasure I will always carry in my heart. I miss her so dearly. I can still feel her rose-and-lilac hugs as she held me closely against her soft breast, and hear her slow Southern drawl.

Warm memories comfort me still. Old-fashioned oatmeal cooked in a little battered tin saucepan, which was then served steaming hot with a generous pat of butter, brown sugar, and real cream that was poured from a little yellow pitcher decorated with colorful flowers.

Growing up I spent most of my summers at Gramma's house, and every Sunday we went to her Baptist church. Sitting next to her, I would draw or write notes to Dear Dr. Richardson, her pastor. His wife once told Gramma that he loved my musings and kept them in a box on his bureau.

I have been reading in Guideposts some uplifting stories of faith about answered prayers. They remind me of Gramma reading similar stories to me when I was a child, sprawled on her big bed, hugging her down pillows to my body, nestling my face into the cool cotton, and breathing in the lingering scent of rose and lavender.

I can see her so clearly, blue eyes sparkling through her glasses, soft aged hands holding this little magazine full of stories of God's love. I can hear her strong voice with a slight quiver of age as she read to me, periodically admonishing me to "keep still a bit" as I fidgeted in youthful exuberance.

Gramma's home was the only place I felt safe and loved. She would read me scriptures from the Bible, and I always asked her to read about the plagues in Exodus. I found them to be the most exciting. Sitting on the chaise in her bedroom, I loved snuggling up to her with my head resting in the warm hollow of her shoulder.

With her worn old Bible in her lap and glasses low on her nose, she read to me and created some of my most special childhood memories. After reading she would take off her glasses with a ceremonial click as she folded them, and she would explain what she had just read. Then to accentuate her point, she would replace her glasses and reread certain verses emphasizing the key message. She had such reverence and unshakeable faith in God's word.

What a precious gift of faith she bestowed on me. I may get discouraged, even angry with the cards dealt to me, but eventually I am able to turn to God and His word for comfort. This morning's thought was quite appropriate. God created the obstacles, which discourage us; He also gave us the power to overcome them.

After Gramma passed, Annie would often pray to her for advice and comfort, flipping through the pages of Gramma's tenderly worn Bible and feeling Gramma's love and presence deep within her.

Annie believed Gramma's spirit was with the Lord and that that spirit was now forever part of the universe.

It is comforting to personalize prayer, to believe that the spirits of our departed loved ones are somehow looking over us, that a part of that spirit remains within us as an extension of the Holy Spirit. Don't we often feel that the spirit of someone we love is watching over us? Ironically, sometimes our actions are guided by this belief with the same strength as our faith in God.

I just spent some quiet time with my Bible. It was the one Gramma used for Sunday school and it means so much to me. She has notes written throughout, and I can almost hear her voice as she reads aloud the verses with vibrant expression, tinged with her gentle Southern drawl.

Smiling now, a full forty years later, I remember my precious Gramma and the magical times at her house. Gramma, the blessing of her, her Bible, her faith, and our treasured times together have sustained and forever enriched my life. Her faith that she passed on to me has saved my life so many times. I was trying to find passages about what heaven may be like. The "Kingdom of Heaven," for example—does it refer to the rule of heaven over earth? I need to call Gramma for references, but of course that is not possible.

Or perhaps the "Kingdom of Heaven" is earthly, organic, manifested in glory on the earth, in the beauty of nature? Flipping through Gramma's Bible, I came across this passage with a large arrow penciled next to it:

Once, on being asked by the Pharisees when the kingdom of God would come, Jesus replied, "The coming of the kingdom of God is not something that can be observed, nor will people say, 'Here it is,' or 'There it is,' because the kingdom of God is in your midst." (Luke 17:20)

My faith is being tried by many ordeals we are facing now. We are facing yet another bleak winter counting pennies and barely making it. Glenn's spirits have taken a nosedive. Evenings spent with Glenn, half dozing in the recliner, spacing out on forgettable television shows, while I sit beside him in my chair reading, taping old movies, or with mindless phone calls. Glenn, tiring of the endless monotony of no work and money woes, escaped into armchair sailing, reading about adventures of cruise live-aboards.

I learned from those sleepless nights with the tear-sodden pillow, trying to hide my fear from Glenn and resenting people who could work, even friends who were succeeding. I was absorbed in anxiety that threatened to suffocate me.

Finally talking to God late one sleepless night, I handed that awful burden over to Him, trying to fully trust in Him. I had wasted so many precious days and weeks, worrying. After all, we were together and I was in a healthy period. To see Glenn so deflated, just plain tired and frustrated, questioning his value as a man, and a provider. How hard I tried to make him realize that his worth wasn't related to a job or money.

Work didn't pick up for a while, but after that night our lives changed. We were laughing again. I was singing in the shower. We made it through that winter with God carrying the mantel of our anxiety.

Annie was many things, all in the same person: a poet who loved words and a great storyteller, irreverent and spiritual at the same time. She fought so many battles wearing her armor of faith, yet she also had the wisdom to know when to surrender and let her belief in the strength and mercy of her Lord pull her through indescribable agony.

Her most favorite Bible passage of all time, the one that sustained her and gave her the most hope came from Isaiah (40:28–31):

"Have you not known? Have you not heard? The Lord is the Everlasting God, the Creator of the ends of the earth. He does not faint or grow weary; His understanding is unsearchable. He gives power to the faint, and strengthens the powerless. Even youths will faint and be weary, and the young will fall exhausted; but those who wait for the Lord shall renew their strength, they shall mount up with wings like eagles, they shall run and not be weary, they shall walk and not faint."

This is one reason why I have titled our joint work *On Eagle's Wings,* because it seemed the perfect expression for the combination of courage and surrender that such a high flight requires—an individual must initiate movement, yet have the simultaneous ability to be buffeted from below by winds of a higher nature.

After Gramma passed, the life-giving faith that Gramma had bestowed in Annie saw her through some of her most trying times. She never preached, that certainly wasn't Annie—but she still influenced many people by being such an example of the power that faith gave her. In time she accepted Gramma's passing, although for the longest time she did not want to see—was not ready to see—her house, which still remained in Annie's extended family.

I can no longer parry excuses not to see Gramma's house. I am torn about this. I have never been there since she left, wanting to leave my vision unmolested.

It was a nostalgic ride down Roland Avenue with those magnificent three- to four-story turn-of-the-century mansions. These beautiful homes, built to house large families, were made of wood, stone, or brick with multitiered roofs.

I looked around the old neighborhood as we drove to Gramma's. A huge lump was in my throat as we pulled up in front. The white clapboard house that I remembered was now painted nutmeg, but the green shutters were still there.

I got out of the car with some trepidation but forged on ahead. There was the gate. My heart caught as I touched this memory-laden piece of yesterday. Gazing up to the front porch, I could see Gramma standing there, arms open in welcome, eyes dancing. Oh Gramma, to clang that gate and walk up those steps.

I could barely hold on. I went on through the old narrow storm door that still sticks and entered the narrow little hallway with wooden steps winding upstairs with the knobbed wooden banister. There was a musty smell, missing only lavender and roses. I opened the next wooden door with its shaky knob. The little mirror on the left wall was still there, but oh my, then what a shock! The dining room was now Melissa's paper-piled, computer- and fax-filled office, and Grampa's room was now a huge modern kitchen.

I closed my eyes for a needed retreat into my memory pictures of how it was. I remember a warm, comforting hideaway for me in a room with a long, thick rose-colored curtain that was the stage curtain for plays that I made up with my cousin Stephen, who with his family was now living in Gramma's house. Little bookshelves were recessed into the walls and lined with pungent smelling old books, family pictures, and little mementos. I can still see every item, run my hands over the books, some from Daddy's boyhood, such as Winnie the Pooh, The Raggedy Man, *and the rhymes of childhood that Gramma used to read to me, such as "Little Orphan Annie's come to our house to stay, to wash the cups 'n saucers and put the plates away." Maybe this was where my love for old books began.*

The little pink bathroom has gone. Pull the stubborn old wood door open, and you are now greeted by a warm rose glow. The skinny tall window by the toilet looks out onto the wood latticed porch, over the yard and the hedges to the sidewalk. I sat my warm fanny on the cold porcelain tub with its narrow hooked chrome spigot and little rubber stopper on a chain. A China angel was sitting on a flowered soap dish. I leaned down by the window and peered out, remembering.

Then I steeled myself and walked into Gramma's bedroom, which was now a dining room. Again the movie in my mind would not allow the present rose-painted and papered room to record.

Instead, the floorboard creaked as I entered. I threw my coat on Gramma's four-poster bed. My younger image reflected in her dressing bureau mirror that dominated the front wall. A little phone table with the old heavy black phone sat beside the pink chair.

My eyes traveled happily around her room, past the living room door, open as always, to the French doors leading to the side porch. Her desk was packed with family pictures, cubbyholes were jammed with papers, and there was the pink blotter and paperweight displaying a picture of the Baptist church inside. Long flowered curtains hung from the three tall bay windows that provided a view of the Franke house next door and the corner railing of the porch.

I pictured Gramma's blue velvet cushioned rocker and her round, wooden Queen Anne table, usually scattered with a few books. A metal floor lamp with a four-cornered shade stood beside her chaise lounge that had a multicolored lap throw over the side. A little bookshelf held her Bible and morning devotional reading.

Opening the door onto Gramma's porch brought a flood of memories and echoes of footfalls. My eyes filled with tears and hurt gripped my chest as my throat tightened. I sat on those wide graceful steps gazing out at the familiar scene of 500 Woodlawn Avenue. The narrow concrete path, bordered by gardens on either side, led to the sidewalk. Voices from a houseful of kids drifted from a wood timbered and stone home, one of many beautiful old homes across the treelined street. I know every patch of sidewalk around all these blocks. Down the alleyways, my mind traveled back in time. Oh Gramma, how I miss you still. Sobs from deep within me rise unbidden and uncontrolled.

I could write a book of memories of my visits, when her home and her loving, generous, warm spirit would surround and comfort me. I spent much of my childhood summers at Gramma's house. The closeness of this bond, her influence and her love, were a most welcome respite during a childhood laced with confusion and pain.

I was afraid that seeing her home changed and redecorated would somehow cloud or taint the images I have cherished, but I found to my relief that I could block out the "now" and return to the pictures in my mind that are indelible and carved on my life stone forever.

The love and laughter that filled her home remains as warm and snug in my heart as it always will for as long as I live.

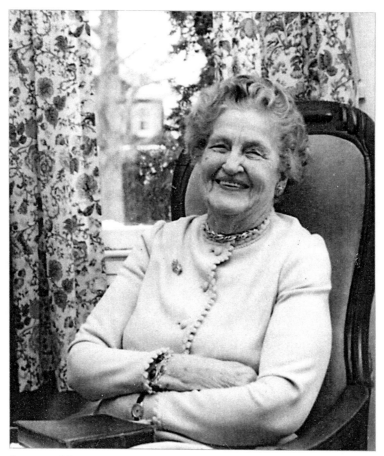

Gramma at home

CHAPTER SIX

Come in and Make Yourself at Home

※⁂※

ANOTHER ONE OF ANNIE'S marvelous coping skills for battling her lifelong health challenges was the care and devotion she gave to animals. Annie loved all kinds of animals: wild, domestic, injured, sick, those in full health, those with an endearing personality, and those with a personality that "only a mother could love." One might think that a passion such as this would be a burden for the other member of a relationship, but Glenn shared Annie's love of animals—together they were truly two peas in a pod . . . two peas plus the extended menagerie they kept both inside and outside their cabin, and later when they were aboard their sailboat *Freyja* as well!

Before he and Annie met, Glenn decided that it would be fun to have a goat. He built a large thirty-by-thirty-foot pen and bought an Alpine billy goat with large curved horns and a long white beard and named him Zeek. Since Alpine goats like to climb, Glenn constructed several different levels of platforms in the pen onto which the goat could scamper. Zeek's favorite was the tallest one where he spent most of his time.

Glenn enjoyed playing a wrestling game with Zeek by holding onto his horns and engaging him in a pushing contest. Grabbing his horns was also a good way to keep from getting butted. After several years, Zeek succumbed to bloat, a condition where the stomach twists, thereby cutting off its supply of oxygen. Glenn rushed him to the vet, but during surgery the vet saw that his stomach had already turned black and it was too late to save him.

A few years after Annie and Glenn were married, Annie wanted to get another goat. Even though he was a billy goat, Annie wanted to name him Gert, which was a dubiously affectionate nickname that her mother had acquired from her children. Gert the goat wasn't the playful animal that Zeek had been. He was ornery and a bully. He occasionally found a way out of the pen, and one morning, when Annie needed to pick up more of her meds, Gert, who had escaped from the pen, wouldn't let her leave the cabin. Every time Annie tried to walk out, Gert would charge, butting the door closed. In desperation, Annie finally called Glenn's mother who agreed to pick up and deliver the medications to Annie.

Being advised of the situation with the goat, Annie's mother-in-law came prepared. Armed with a long two-by-four board she wielded like a ninja warrior, and with shrieking war cries, she fought her way down the path to the cabin. Watching safely from a window, Annie was hysterical with laughter. It was quite a comical sight watching this little five-foot-two woman fending off a rampaging goat.

After neighbors down the road reported that Gert had also imprisoned them in their houses, it was decided that Gert had to go. Fortunately for everyone, a farmer in the area was looking for a billy goat for his herd of all female goats. Glenn and Annie were all too happy to donate their goat to the farmer's herd, and Gert was delighted.

Any visit to Annie and Glenn's house would undoubtedly involve an unexpected interaction or several with animals of all varieties. Annie and Glenn were so used to living with their menagerie that they would forget that this was considered a bit out of the ordinary.

There was a time when Annie was in the hospital and Doug, Glenn's childhood friend who had been away for a few years, was coming over to see him. Remembering that Doug enjoyed beer, Glenn ran out to get some after leaving a note on the door that read, "Beer run, in case I'm not back yet, come in and make yourself at home."

When Doug arrived, Glenn wasn't there, so as instructed, Doug went in and sat in a large comfortable looking chair in the addition. All of a sudden his eye caught two baby skunks as they ran out from underneath the chair. That unexpected surprise startled him, but before he had time to react, his attention was taken by the sensation of his ear being played with. He turned around to see a huge raccoon sitting on the back of the chair staring at him. A moment later a ferret, who had been taking a nap under the cushion and was not happy about being sat on, wiggled out from underneath the cushion and, taking revenge, bit him on the butt.

When Glenn arrived home, Doug was waiting for him outside in the front yard.

Annie was much more intentional about introducing visitors to the wonderful world of animals.

> Glenn was at work and I was by myself in the cabin and feeling lonely.
>
> There was a knock on the door, and it was the delivery guy whose intention was simply to deliver the lumber that Glenn had ordered, have the invoice signed, and be on his way.
>
> But oh no, I greeted the young black man in my pj's and robe with uncombed zombie hair. I introduced myself and invited this complete stranger into my house and proceeded to take this bewildered, but very pleasant and polite, young man on a cabin tour, climaxed by dragging him into the raccoon pen out back. I told him about Pepper, our forty-pound Buddha Butt raccoon, but wanted him to meet our baby twins that we had raised practically since birth.
>
> Cajoled into the twins' large, walk-in cage, his weak cries of "I am not touching no raccoon," and

"Where is that big one?" were somewhat reassured when I told him that he was not going to be pounced upon.

I grabbed his hesitant hand and physically propelled his unwilling feet into the enclosed pen of Zuzu and Zorro, all the while soothingly telling him that these "little" guys were only four-month-old orphans raised from four-ounce babies that fit into your palm. "Be very gentle, Henry, they are more scared of you than you are of them," if that were possible! The poor kid, he was really spooked about this whole ordeal with eyes wide as he cautiously and constantly peered around him checking his means of escape.

He was holding one hand on the door jamb as I, holding his other hand, pulled him forward toward the "kids'" sleeping quarters. Zuzu, the braver one, peeked her head through the opening. Henry nearly pulled me over as he backed away posthaste.

"That coon is huge! That ain't no baby!"

"Yes, Henry, she is, so gentle, such a baby, it is okay really. They were hand-raised.... Here, come give me your hand, no really, hold my hand, let her sniff you." With eyes widening, Henry hesitantly but trustingly gave me his hand, and I steered it toward the curious raccoon.

Zuzu sniffed, ears perked forward, then reached a tentative hand toward Henry.

"C'mon, Henry, feel how soft her paws are. Have you ever seen how cool their feet are? They're

like our hands aren't they?" And before he knew what was really happening, he relaxed and was stroking her paws and smiling.

Before Henry left he thanked me for the experience and said he couldn't wait to get home to tell his wife about how he was in a cage with raccoons and actually touched one.

He had reluctantly been forced into an experience by some zany, nature-loving lady who lived in the woods in a real log cabin with a bunch of animals, and he will never forget it.

I then signed his invoice, and he was on his way.

Over the years there were several pet ferrets that lived at the cabin. About ten years into their marriage, Annie and Glenn adopted the first one from a pet store when he was six or seven weeks old. He was given the name Sweeper because he would scoot underneath the furniture and come out looking like a dust ball.

Sweeper was definitely Annie's pet. One of his favorite places to be was snuggled inside the front, hand-warmer pocket of a sweatshirt that Annie was wearing. Keeping him inside the cabin was always a concern, but when he occasionally got out he always came back to the sound of a squeaky toy.

Sweeper had them terribly worried one day when he was nowhere to be found, and after several hours of searching, the whole neighborhood was recruited and armed with squeaky toys in search of Sweeper. While everyone was out searching frantically for him, it seems that Sweeper was safely and happily taking a nap curled up in a drawer in the house.

Tilly was a special ferret and gained notoriety when she crawled inside their computer and made a nest in the hard drive. A panel was missing in the front and the space within apparently looked like a good nesting place—good for nesting but bad for the computer! A repairman was summoned to the cabin and was so amused with the reason for the call that he wrote an article about the ferret, which he submitted to a computer magazine.

His article was published and not only was Annie and Glenn's service bill waved but the broken computer was replaced with a brand-new one, compliments of the magazine.

Blossom and Sassy were skunks that they bought at a pet shop when it was still legal to do so. They were six-to eight-weeks old and had been spayed and de-scented. Skunks are pretty little animals, very affectionate, and can become quite domesticated if adopted when they are still very young.

They always remained a bit skittish, and when a sudden movement or noise startled them they would stomp their feet and turn around and flick their tail at you. Any available lap was a good place for a nap, and they often curled up together to sleep. When they were awake, they spent a lot of time playing with each other. A favorite pastime was checking out what was underneath the furniture. Anything their head could fit under, their body could follow.

Of all of the animals that Glenn and Annie shared their lives with, the species that was the most treasured in their heart was the raccoon, whether wild, rehabilitated, or domesticated.

I'm lying on my swing, covered in a fuzzy blanket with the sun warm on my face. I have just spent the last twenty minutes visiting the raccoons in their condo cages, wrapped up in sixty pounds of warm cuddly coons, and I am reminiscing. I am picturing pulling my sweatshirt hood over my head as I leaned my head and arms into their outdoor condo with one arm around each furry body. Fred leans down from the second floor with his black button nose sniffing expectantly. His liquid eyes were sleepy but intent on my face. His paws reach forward to touch my face with little fingers probing my mouth and nose. Lucy grabs my jacket and thrusts her head down my chest just like when she was a baby. Ethel has hold of my zipper and is trying to chew it off while Fred continues exploring my face. What a blessing this is. I feel so warm and content.

I am reminded of another experience, which still leaves me breathless, humbled, and disbelieving over what happened. It was almost like an out-of-body raccoon experience.

I was awake all night wrapped in a blanket of unutterable back, rib, and now, yahoo, leg agony and was despairing over my total inability to move, stand, or walk!

Then God provided me with the most touching and inspirational experience. I was watching the neighborhood wild raccoons gobble up the last dust from the feeding station that we put out nightly for their dining pleasure. I can't help but smile the whole time I watch their signature antics. Three to four would back up to one pan, literally butting the competition out of their way.

It was just like when you were kids sitting close together, usually on a bench located near some festivity, which of course, required your best behavior. You would cast a sideways mischievous smile with eyes twinkling at your friend. That's all it would take to begin serious butt and thigh pushing. Goal scored if your partner in crime was pushed off or better yet yelled at by an older presence to "Be still!"

As the sky began to lighten, all the coons slowly galumphed off, stopping every few seconds for a quick front paw poking at the ground. You never know where there may be a tasty tidbit that was missed.

Then I caught a movement on the deck and right by the sliding door stood a bear-like mama raccoon with four babies. We had been watching the quads for a week now. Two of them are almost teens, and then wondrously, there are two wee tiny babies that even still have baby fuzz on their heads. The runt is only a bit larger than the length of my hand. The little ones are too young to really have fear so their cues come from Mama.

Then they began climbing the screen. I very painfully and slowly made it to my wheels and was off to the fridge for yogurt and a food drawer for granola. I fixed them a good breakfast. I have been concerned about "Tiny" and whether he was getting enough food. He has an injured back foot and his limp is pronounced. As I approached the door with the goodies in my lap, Mama came forward and touched the screen. I slid the screen back. The noise didn't faze her one bit. I put the two dishes down inches from the open door and the babies all came out from under Gramma's chaise lounge on the little patio. I deliberately placed one yogurt dish right in front of the door, and the two runts claimed it. They were so near, yet so far. My eyes were tear-filled knowing we won't have any babies this year. I could not control myself and my hand, with a mind of its own, reached down from my chair to caress the baby. Tiny stopped chewing for a second and gave me a sideways glance as I was petting him. Then he simply went back to his gourmet treat of yogurt and granola bits. I loved looking at his little, wee feet, excuse for a tail, and little baby fuzz head bordered by tiny black velvet ears. I could barely comprehend that by God's grace I was petting a wild baby raccoon. Mama only gave a precautionary grumble but didn't stop eating. Cursing my physical inability to bend for more than a few seconds, I watched enthralled, grateful, and joyous as they licked their plates clean.

Then with a trill-trill, the babies were beckoned to follow her. Daylight was here, and it was time for bed now. She trotted off with the quads in single file behind her. The teens remained in the lead, Tee, sis of Tiny, came next, and then last limped Tiny. When he got too far behind, it touched me to see his mom circle back and wait for her smallest to catch up.

Precious and ever to be remembered, this was a Kodak image of Mama and all four of her babies following single file across the bridge. I strained to see where they were heading. They crossed the bridge over the stream, heading to the back property.

This was a miracle. How do I get to have the privilege of communicating with these darling, remarkable creatures, to actually stroke a wild baby's back?

Before they were married, when Glenn first moved Annie into his cabin to take care of her, they also brought back Maude, the baby raccoon that had been given to her by her stepsister after Annie's surgery. Annie had always been a caretaker for orphaned or injured animals, but it was Annie that now needed the care. Nevertheless they weren't about to abandon this baby raccoon, so Maude became another passenger in the truck heading back to New Jersey with Glenn, Annie, and Elka.

Glenn built a cage around a large section of woods with an enclosed run leading from the cage to their bedroom window on the second floor of the cabin. This gave Maude access to the outdoors as well as to the house.

Baby raccoons need to be adopted before they are six to eight weeks old or they have little chance of becoming domesticated. Maude had been acquired after this period of time, and as she got older her wild side became more evident. She became increasingly aggressive until one day she stood at the top of the stairs, raised up like a mama grizzly bear protecting her young, and wouldn't let Glenn up the stairs. That is when she was given her freedom but would often return for food that was always left out for her.

Still, Annie wanted a raccoon. Her family had a pet raccoon named Robbie when she was a child, and she developed a special love for the little masked bandit. Through a local pet store, they heard about a mail-order company in Minnesota where there was a farm that raised raccoons to sell for their pelts and training coon dogs. They had a runt of the litter they were willing to sell and ship to Philadelphia. One of the flight crew fell in love with the five-week-old infant raccoon and held him on her lap for most of the flight.

Annie and Glenn had already decided on the name Pepper for their new pet because it was a unisex name and they didn't know what they were getting. It is almost impossible to tell the sex of a raccoon when it is still so young. The vet thought that it was a girl, but one day when Pepper's "belly button" sprung a leak they realized that they had a little boy. They were happy with this discovery because male raccoons usually aren't as aggressive as females, who are born with a fierce instinct to protect their young.

Their first day at home with baby Pepper was delightful as they watched him investigate his new surroundings. Annie and Glenn took turns holding and feeding him a bottle. He was an active, curious little guy and a great source of entertainment.

After a tiring day they hoped that Pepper would sleep well that night. They had prepared a little crate for him right next to their bed, said good night to him, and climbed into bed. Being in a strange place and in need of comfort, he cried and scratched until Annie was so desperate to sleep that she brought the little masked baby into their bed. That was the last night Pepper was ever put in his crate.

Raccoons are by nature nocturnal, but he pretty much adapted to their schedule. Pepper would often leave their bed for a few hours in the middle of the night to explore the house but would be back in bed again before morning. When he was chilly, he would snuggle in behind Glenn's knees, but if it was hot, he would push their heads off of their pillow and claim it as his own with no regard or concern for it having already been occupied. He often found great delight in ripping open a pillow, pulling out the stuffing, and tossing it around the bed. Pillows were frequently replaced.

His diet included scrambled eggs, yogurt, cereal, fruit, and dry dog food. Meat was never part of his diet because it makes raccoons aggressive.

One day Annie and Glenn set out for Philadelphia to visit Annie's family for the day. Left at home alone without supervision, Pepper took full advantage of his freedom. After returning home and before dealing with the full scope of the cleanup, Annie first went to the bathroom and was surprised but had to laugh to see it looking like "mischief night," as it had been decorated with toilet paper that was draped all over in interesting designs.

The kitchen, however, being the main target of the invasion, looked like a war zone. It was hard to believe that one raccoon could create damage equal to a military raid. A canister of flour had been tipped over, and flour was spilled on the counters and floor with incriminating white coon tracks leading away from the crime scene. Cereal was scattered about, and the water was left running full force in the sink. Cabinets had been invaded and rifled through, and while Pepper had been seeking some unknown special delight, he had tossed aside many of the products. The attack on the refrigerator was relentless. The door was standing open, and the contents, pulled out for inspection, were now disassembled on the floor. A carton of eggs had toppled out, and while some of the yolks stayed intact, the ones that didn't joined the whites that had crept their way under the refrigerator. Other incriminating evidence was found in a pile of mashed potatoes that were indented with raccoon paw prints looking like the impression of a child's handprint in plaster. Milk and orange juice cartons lay sideways on the floor, with their liquid making colorful rivers across the brick and damming up at the edge of the braided living room rug. Lids had been removed from storage containers that were under investigation so that their contents could be sampled. Pepper had a sweet tooth and so, to top off his meal, he opened a bottle of Peppermint Schnapps. The sweet taste appealed to him, but it seems he wasn't so good at holding his liquor. Annie and Glenn had to laugh at his slightly drunken state. He kept putting his hands over his eyes, and Annie thought perhaps this was his attempt to stop the room from spinning.

After that incident, unless he was being supervised, Pepper was confined to the second floor of the cabin, from which he could also access his outdoor living space. Whenever guests were in the house, he was kept upstairs and then only by request was he brought down for a short visit. As affectionate as Pepper was with Annie and Glenn, he was wary of other people. Only a few were able to hold him, but he was tolerant of letting others touch him if Annie or Glenn were holding him. The runt of the litter grew to be quite a large raccoon weighing forty pounds, and in spite of his weight, Annie was able to carry him. Pepper would put his arms around her neck while she supported his bottom and carried him around like a mother would carry a child in a sling.

Our reputation for nurturing injured or infant wildlife was widespread, so it wasn't unusual one day when we found eight baby skunks in a box at our front door. They were still infants and of course we brought them in. Pepper was quite curious about the new babies, and a few days after their arrival he cornered one of them in the craft room. The scared little skunk instinctively defended himself, and Pepper got sprayed.

The scent of skunk spray from a distance is like a drop in the ocean compared with the potency of a close, fresh spray, which is so powerful that it makes your eyes burn and water. Even after washing Pepper numerous times and continuously airing out the craft room with fans, it took a month for the smell to dissipate enough to where the room could be used. The offending baby and her siblings were quickly moved into a pen outdoors.

The little skunks got used to being handled and enjoyed the interaction with humans. Their fur was soft and silky, and it was fun to play with the babies.

When they were infants, they were fed puppy formula and human baby rice cereal until they had enough teeth to chew. Their diet was then changed to scrambled eggs, granola bars, and cat food.

Other than being raised by humans, this litter was different because of their unusual markings. It was pretty clear that an albino skunk that had been spotted in the area had parented this litter. One of the babies had normal skunk markings on his head, but the rest of his body was totally white. Another was all white except for the black leggings and boots it looked like he was wearing on all four legs and feet. A black diamond on the chest of another was the only contrast to his all-white body. Only two of the eight babies had normal skunk markings.

After being with us for two months, the skunks had grown bigger, and their pen was moved about a half block from the cabin. They continued to be fed but their door was left ajar. We were offered money for them, but we had always intended to return the skunks to the wild when they were old enough to survive on their own.

The litter gradually investigated more and more of the area but would return to the pen for food. As they became more comfortable with the surrounding woods, they depended less on being fed and adapted to their natural life as wild creatures. Eventually the pen was abandoned.

An abandoned pen meant success—if an animal could be rehabilitated to that degree. Otherwise they were welcome to stay. In the aviary that Glenn built, Annie and Glenn cared for screech owls, crows, sea gulls, and other injured birds that were brought to them. In the summer tourist season of Cape May, traffic is increased and birds are hit by cars and suffer from shock or broken wings. Even after careful treatment, some birds are just sick, disabled, or too young to be released back into nature. Annie once tamed a crow, for example, that would not have made it in the wild again after having been injured, but it became a good pet.

Their close friend, Steve, had a degree in biology and had also been a vet assistant. Although Steve took in injured or orphaned wildlife, much of it he handed over to Annie and Glenn because his interest was in reptiles and he was considered one of the top authorities in the country on turtles. Annie and Glenn preferred creatures with fur.

When Glenn found two brown water snakes in the corner of their pond, he called Steve and told him that he was very welcome to them. Steve came over and went into the pond barefoot, wearing just shorts, and retrieved five snakes. Snakes were one thing that Glenn did not like.

They had a wonderful friendship and working relationship, trading favors in many ways. Steve often cared for the critters that Annie and Glenn couldn't take aboard when they later bought a sailboat and would escape on an odyssey. In return, Glenn built cages to house the many creatures that lived on Steve's property.

Steve named his rescue and sanctuary, "New Jersey Nature," and Annie and Glenn's was "Nature's Way." Annie became the education consultant for both New Jersey Nature and Nature's Way, taking critters to schools and other organizations, and in this way recovering a part of her originally intended vocation of teaching children. I think Annie also found great satisfaction in taking care of injured animals as a way of passing on the kindnesses of care she had herself received over the years from so many talented doctors, nurses, and physical therapists.

Nature's Way is absolutely bursting at the seams with life beyond our wildest dreams.

Glenn and I are caring for sixteen baby raccoons. "Johnny" is with his sisters, "Panda 1" and "Panda 11."

And then there is "Midget" and "J.J.," the infant saved by a friend four weeks ago, so wild, so scared, so adorable. I have gained her trust and she always greets me now. She is bunking with "Wee One," the smallest of the pack and one from Steve's wild horde. The "Magnificent Seven" were also brought by Steve and are occupying three front pens.

When houses are being renovated, sometimes nests of raccoon babies are found. They are getting better now about trying to trap the mother so she can be placed with the babies and take care of them. Then they are all put in a pen and released together. Otherwise the babies would die if not taken in by a human who cares and has the knowledge to raise them until they can be released.

Everywhere you look there is a furry little masked cutie. We are in coon heaven.

Whoops, almost forgot our two girls, Pooka and Zuzu.

Baby raccoons are our little prayers not just because we dearly wanted wee babies to care for but because of the inner smiles, comfort, and release that just their being brings to us.

To add to the show we also have five baby opossums, two precious skunks, and one blind house finch. Peter Finch has been with us for five months now. All of our new critters, of course, are in addition to our domestic crew. Over the years we have had raccoons, swans, geese, ducks, possums, skunks, rabbits, squirrels, a fawn, turtles, a variety of birds, barn owls, sea gulls, a kestrel, a red-tailed hawk, and Curley, a screech owl who consciously does not flex his talons when I handle him so I don't have to use gauntlets.

They all get named whether they are with us for a short time or a lifetime. It is fun finding names that seem to fit. I remember Fred, Ethel, and Lucy, our triplet baby raccoons that we had for a season.

We aren't licensed rehabbers, but the fish and game people still bring us animals to care for. There

*are just more animals that need care than people
who are willing to care for them.*

Annie had often seen a young dog tied by wire to a post in the middle of a small field about a hundred feet from a rundown-looking house. She had heard that the couple living in the house had severe drug problems and that they would lose a dog every few months. The dogs would either run away or were killed on the highway not far from their house.

This sad-looking dog was tethered to prevent him from running off, and there was no food or water in sight. Very concerned, she started bringing water to him. After several days of checking up on him and seeing that he was being badly neglected, Annie couldn't stand it any longer, so she untied him and brought him home with her.

He was a short-haired, medium-size dog with fur that was various shades of tan except for a darker colored back. His muzzle and the tips of his ears were black. It was obvious that he was badly in need of a bath, a good meal, and a lot of love.

The vet thought he was about a year old and gave him his shots and an exam. Annie named him Tippy and wasn't sure if that was because he had one ear that tipped over or because he had a white tip on the end of his tail. She figured that either reason worked.

Several months later a man showed up at her door claiming that she had stolen his dog and demanded him back. Annie paled in size to this large, angry man, but she stood up to him hoping that he couldn't see her shaking.

She threatened to call the police and the humane society if he didn't get off of her property. He never came back.

Glenn had some mending to do on the fence that enclosed almost half of their four acres, and before it was finished Tippy would find a way out and go for a "walkabout." He always came back except for one time when he had been gone for several hours, and worried, Annie and Glenn went looking for him. They found him on the road, slowly limping his way back home. They immediately took him to the vet. He had many cuts that needed stitching and bruises but no broken bones. They weren't sure what had caused the injuries, but they suspected that he might have been beaten. Tippy was very sore and received lots of tender loving care while he was healing.

After that Tippy was put on a run when he was outside until Glenn could find and fix the places on the fence where he had gotten out—at the same time, Tippy seemed to have reached the conclusion independently that he wanted to stay. He knew he had a good home and had no desire to leave.

When Annie and Glenn became sailors, Tippy loved being on the boat. He was happy standing at the bow with the wind blowing his ears back. Whenever Annie and Glenn would sail to the Chesapeake, Tippy would be their first mate. They would have to go ashore every day to let him have a run and do his business. During one of the landings they pulled into an uninhabited island and let Tippy off the leash. Tippy took off, and when they looked up they saw him running side by side with a red fox. The two of them raced around together for a while, and eventually the fox ran off into the brush and Tippy returned to Annie and Glenn. They enjoyed watching this brief friendship between their dog and a fox.

Tippy was often at Annie's side when she would write in her journal. He was a very lucky dog to have been rescued from a sad life in favor of one that was filled with love and adventure.

Another spring morning, Annie got a call from a friend who told her that she had found a parrot on her bird feeder and asked if Annie could take him.

Of course, Annie was never known to turn down any creature that was in need, so Mac was introduced into their family that already included two dogs, numerous cats, a rabbit, two possums, two skunks, a goat, a ferret, and a raccoon, not to mention the wild bunch who were in their rehab care.

Mac was a ruby-throated, yellow-crowned Amazon parrot. He arrived with a strange vocabulary that led them to believe that he had spent time in a barnyard. No one knew how long he had been on his own, but it was thought that he might have found refuge in a barn over the winter. His imitations included a chicken, duck, blue jay, and crow, but the funniest one was whinnying like a horse.

Annie and Glenn spent most of their time in the "addition" but Mac's cage had been relegated to the living room because he was so loud. It never failed to make them laugh when he came out with one of his imitations, especially the whinny when you could just swear that there was a horse in the living room.

He would also say the expected "hello" to anyone who would enter the room and had perfected the wolf whistle.

Living at the cabin, he also learned to imitate a sea gull and a squeaky toy. It was amusing when Mac would do his impression of a squeaky toy and the ferret would run circles around the bottom of the hanging cage trying to find it.

When Annie and Glenn first got Mac, Annie took him to the vet to get his wings clipped. Flight feathers grow back to their full length two or three times a year so it is never permanent, but proper clipping will keep the bird from being able to fly away until the feathers grow back. Annie left the vet with Mac on her shoulder, and on her way to the car Mac flew up into the nearest tree . . . so much for the proper clipping. Annie hurried back into the vet's for help in retrieving him. The staff all came out and eventually got Mac back and reclipped his too capable wings.

Mac was definitely Annie's bird. He would ride around on her shoulders and give her kisses on the cheek. Even though it was Glenn who took care of his cage and kept him with food and water, his only thank-you was a bite on the hand and his curved beak could easily draw blood.

It was estimated that Mac was about three or four years old when they got him, and parrots typically live for about forty to fifty years. Mac had been living with Annie and Glenn for ten years when he developed an upper respiratory infection. The vet gave him medicine but warned them that parrots usually do not recover from this type of ailment. Two days later Annie and Glenn tearfully buried Mac.

Annie was very sad after losing Mac and missed having a bird, so she went to a pet store and came home with a cockatiel. A cockatiel is a small Australian parrot about the size of a cardinal but with a longer tail. They are gray and white with perfectly placed round red spots on their cheeks and a yellow mask running across their eyes.

Annie named him Fred. Fred only had one thing to say and that was "Oh my God," and he repeated it often as if to make up for the lack of his limited vocabulary.

Fred's cage hung from a pulley system in the middle of the living room. This allowed the cage to be lowered for cleaning and allowed Annie to get Fred in and out of his cage. The rest of the time, Fred was hoisted up and out of danger from the cats that showed an unhealthy interest in Fred.

The cats were often cleared from the room, allowing Fred to fly around, free of danger.

Glenn walked into the cabin one evening after visiting Annie during one of her hospital stays and found the cage door open and no Fred. There were feathers everywhere but no sign of poor Fred. It was surmised that somehow Fred managed to unlatch his cage door and flew out. The rest can only be unpleasantly imagined.

Returning to the hospital the next day, Glenn had the reluctant duty of telling Annie about the tragic demise of Fred. Annie was horrified and cried. After a few minutes, however, through her tears she started to laugh and said, "Oh Glenn, poor Fred, I can just see him getting caught by one of the cats and squawking, 'Oh my God, oh my God.'"

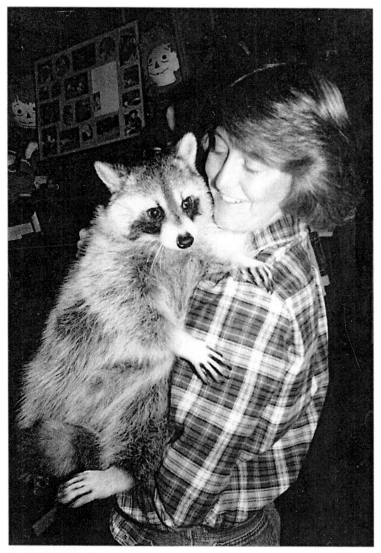

That's a lot of raccoon

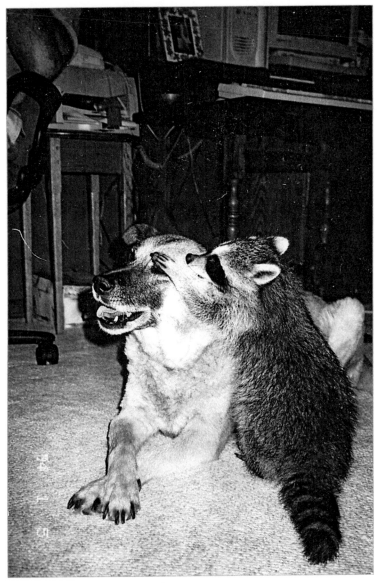

Pepper and Tippy playing together

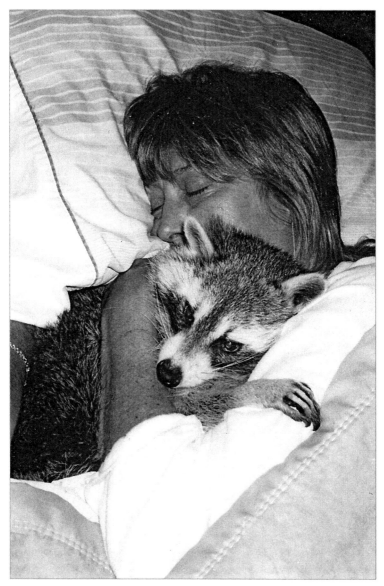

Annie sleeping with Pepper

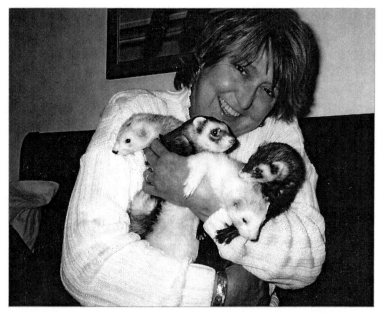

How many ferrets can Annie hold?

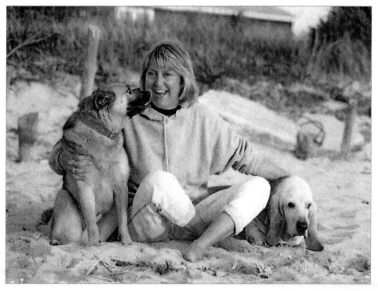

Annie with her buddies, Tippy and Scupper

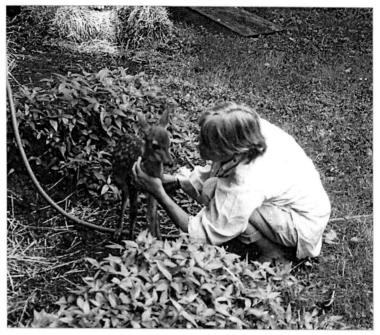

Just one of the many animals being cared for at Nature's Way

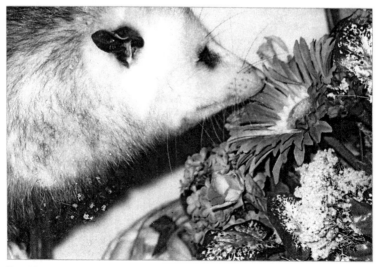

Freckles the possum taking time to smell the flowers

CHAPTER SEVEN

All Aboard the Christmas Express!

✖

IN 1984, WHEN ANNIE WAS 36, she was working for the school system and tutoring pregnant teenagers. In those days, once a girl started to "show" she would not be allowed to attend school so she received her education at home. One cold December morning, Annie went to see her new assignment, a thirteen-year-old girl soon to be a mother. Arriving at her destination, Annie saw a small, dilapidated house with badly peeling paint. The roof looked like it could not prevent even a moderate drizzle from leaking into the house, and the front steps were rotting in several places so that you had to choose your footing carefully. Littering the front porch were useless household objects—there was either no time to clean up these items, or the owner of the house had succumbed to the idea of being surrounded with junk as a way of living. A rusted-out car sat on the front lawn looking like it had found its final resting place.

Annie knocked and waited long enough to wonder—almost hope—that she had the wrong house. Then her new student opened the door. Annie looked at the girl with her swollen belly and saw she was but a child herself. How could she possibly be ready to be a mother?

Inside the house, the lighting was dim as there was no electricity. It was chilly as well; one could smell the kerosene from the heater that provided the only source of warmth. Smoke from the heater tinted the panes of glass in the windows with a film, diminishing the sun's efforts to brighten the room.

The girl showed Annie to a cluttered table where she hastily cleared a pot of noodles that had evidently been cooked for breakfast. Once space had been created for their lesson, the two sat down and opened an assignment book. Annie's attention was drawn to a young child, between the stages of sitting and walking, who was sitting on the floor entertaining himself by tearing pieces from a cardboard box.

Glancing further around the room, Annie had the striking realization that although four children lived in this house, there were no toys anywhere. In addition, the pregnant teen, with no means of supporting herself, would soon be adding an infant to the household. The teen's single mother worked for minimum wage, and there simply wasn't enough money for the luxury of toys. Just being able to feed and clothe her family and keep a roof over their heads was all that her meager paycheck would allow.

Annie's heart went out to these children, who had nothing to play with except whatever they could devise with their imagination. Life would be hard enough—but to never be able to enjoy one's childhood? Annie could not bear that thought or the realization of how the mother must feel not being able to give her children a single gift for Christmas.

Christmas had always been Annie's favorite time of year. She would plan for months ahead, making lists and perusing catalogues for just the right gift for everyone. Oftentimes Annie and Glenn would craft their gift by hand out of Glenn's exquisite woodworking, with Annie applying the finishing touches by paintbrush. Annie loved making something personal for those she loved, and loved giving something of herself.

At holiday time, Glenn and Annie's cabin was warm and glowed with decorations. The tree was adorned with an overload of brightly colored lights and sentimental ornaments, many of them little raccoons that looked right at home sitting in the branches. Every doorway and window was outlined with festive lights. Outside, Christmas lights framed the roof and windows, and a large Santa and snowman stood watch. Glenn had developed his own method of decorating the trees outside of their wooded property. First he would straighten out a long string of lights and gather them as a cowboy would gather his rope and then, holding tightly onto the plug, he would toss the entire string of lights as high as he could up into a tree. Where they landed is where they stayed. The effect was always interesting, and Annie and Glenn would sit snug in their cabin, looking across the pond at the unpredictable designs being duplicated in the water, trying to visualize forms in them as one would when gazing at clouds.

There is a festive yet restful mood in our cabin home as darkness comes. The lights outside are glowing gaily. The waterfall and bridge are lit at night with strings of lights that reflect on the ice-covered pond. Lights around the arbor and from the shop give the feeling of a winter wonderland.

Patches of snow hug the pines, and the green and red lights give off a muted glow. A wreath of lights is next to the door, and the whole porch and edges of the roof are outlined in multicolored lights.

Lights, lights, lights, oh how they illuminate our spirit. Our Christmas tree is glowing in front of me. My favorite sight is the multicolored reflections of lights in every dark window. Green garlands with twinkling white lights surround Gramma's large mirror over my bed in the addition and are reflected in the windows in front of me. The gleaming white ceramic nativity scene is placed on the windowsill with little winged angels flying overhead, suspended by invisible fishing line. Candles on each side give the whole scene a peaceful glow.

Treasured Santas, each representing a Christmas past, have their own special place. It is truly a Christmas room.

Thoughts of our Jimmy Buffet Christmas tribute always bring a giggle. One Christmas when

I was bed bound, Glenn, with his eyes twinkling, had me close my eyes, and then with a flick of a switch he said, "Now open them." And what to my wondering eyes should appear but a light-trimmed Caribbean scene out by the pond, complete with pink flamingos, a four-foot palm tree, and two life-size dolphins!

Then comes the quiet, reflective mood of the day after Christmas, which is infused with love that was showered upon me on Christmas day. It was a wondrous day with long-anticipated surprises. Glenn, my precious Santa, again put such thought and obvious care into each gift. He prided himself on not taking the easy route, choosing not to give me one thing that I asked for but instead, substituting my suggestions with well-thought-out mischievous and endearing gifts.

Things, yes, and as is usually the case, most "things" are forgotten. It is the memory of how his thoughtfulness makes me feel, knowing the effort and love that went into each dear gift that makes it special.

The stark contrast between the kind of Christmases that Annie and Glenn shared and the Christmas that awaited impoverished families like the one her student belonged to was unacceptable to Annie. While there were organizations and charities for many causes, Annie soon discovered that there was absolutely nothing in the whole area that would help these families have a brighter Christmas.

"Well, something has to be done about this," Annie said to herself, and in addition to money of her own, she called upon us, her friends and family, to donate ten dollars each for her cause. She used the money that she collected that year and purchased gifts and clothing for the family of her student, leaving them at the family's door with a note from Santa stating "All aboard the Christmas Express!" If the student suspected Annie as the cause of her family's recent benefaction, she didn't mention it, nor did Annie volunteer that information. Annie simply loved Christmas with the heart of a child. She couldn't think of a better way to celebrate Christmas than to experience the joy of giving.

The next year Annie expanded her Christmas Express by reaching out to the community. She got newspapers to print stories about the number of underprivileged people in their own communities who were barely making it on their own. Most of them were single-parent families.

As Annie told local reporters, "These gifts are far more than a present in a box. They give individuals hope by letting them know that their community cares about them."

Inspired by her student, Annie became especially interested in teens from abused, neglected, or otherwise dysfunctional families.

Everybody thinks of little children, but they often forget the teens. And for them, it's just as important, if not more so, to have Christmas presents because they are at the age when they're making many important decisions. I refer to the children in this age group as "forgotten." It's easy for strangers to

*buy a stuffed animal for a young child, but people
don't know what to get a teenager. And so these
kids, aged thirteen to eighteen, end up being the
ones who do not have a Christmas. Yet it is these
very children who are going to be our citizens ten
years down the line.*

Annie worked closely with a local Cape May agency, Cape Counseling, to locate these teens, many of whom were in "safe homes" where they had been placed following abuse or other domestic problems. The Coalition Against Rape and Abuse (CARA) was another one of her sources for finding young women who needed help. Annie knew that kids brought up in poverty often have low self-esteem. But she also knew that if these kids felt there were people who cared about them, even if they didn't know them, that their spirits—and their prospects—could be brightened immeasurably.

It was the spirit of the season that held Annie in such thrall, and which she so badly wanted to share. Annie was adamant that Christmas Express was not just asking for money, but that it was actually making a difference in the lives of people. Penny for penny, all of the money collected was used for gifts, toys for children who, because they had never had anything, didn't expect much. A seven-year-old boy, for example, asked for a Matchbox car, a dollar toy, while a little four-year-old girl asked for a box of crayons.

Donations came to Christmas Express in many ways. Most of the money was accumulated from many people giving a small amount, and Annie was grateful for each and every dollar. But as word of mouth spread about Christmas Express, there would sometimes come a windfall from an organization or a business that gave a large donation. Many store owners or managers whom Annie had befriended were then able to stretch that money by offering generous discounts. And of course there were the sales—which Annie and Glenn took full advantage of. As Glenn told me, "When you're buying fifteen hairdryers, a good sale price makes all the difference!"

So many heartwarming stories this year!

A ten-year-old boy and his father made two trips into a bank where a donation box had been placed. They were carrying jars full of pennies, nickels, and dimes. The boy had been saving for a whole year to buy a cassette deck but had seen the article in the paper about Christmas Express and decided to give us his entire savings saying, "Some kids don't have nothing. I guess they need it more than I do."

Two weeks before the Big Day, we had a request for nine bikes from a group home for teenagers in Woodbine. There were currently nine teens at the home, ages twelve to sixteen, who were making their own family that year. We were almost out of money but we were determined to get those bikes. We called all of the bike rentals and shops, but no one could help us. One of the Express helpers who did legwork for us was headed for her hairdresser and made a wrong turn that landed her on an unfamiliar street. Not knowing where she was, she stopped and knocked on the door of a house that had a "dune buggies" sign outside. "Why am I doing this?" she asked herself. The door opened, and Nicholas Elmer, who also restores and repairs bicycles, stood there surrounded by bicycles, all of which had been restored. He only charged us fifty dollars for nine bikes and even offered to deliver them on Christmas Eve. Can you believe that, a man named Nick making special deliveries on Christmas Eve? That's what I call a miracle!

Three days before Christmas, we had a blizzard, the kind we don't get on the coast very often so when one does come you know it means business. We were getting ready for a cozy, inside day when there was a knock on the door of the cabin around 8:00 a.m.

A woman standing there said, "My father told me to come to you. We have twenty special needs children, and we're going to have a party but the toys that we planned for them cannot be delivered through the snow. Do you have anything?"

Just the night before someone had dropped off two large trash bags of winter coats. When we opened the bags there were coats and jackets in excellent condition, some still with tags on them. There were enough for all of the children. Another person had provided a bag of toys that I was also able to give the woman for the children. Another Christmas miracle . . . .

Annie held a special place in her heart for the business owners who would always hear her out even if they couldn't give anything at the moment. But they usually did give, and give generously! She told me once about the time when a seven-year-old's bike was stolen two days before Christmas. At 11:00 p.m. Christmas Eve, she went to Bruce Hale, a local shop owner, and he donated a bike.

Another time Annie got a call about eight children whose only parent had just been taken to jail, and the children were staying with their twenty-one-year-old sister.

> *I had already spent all the money. I didn't know what I was going to do. I called the At Home Shop and my friend there made sure they had all the home supplies they needed. I also called Tommy Markle of the Mimi Shop in Stone Harbor. He's a hard-driving businessman, but he's got a heart of gold. He told me, "Bring them all in here and I'll make sure they all have a Christmas outfit."*
>
> *The owner of a hardware store took a cart and went down the aisles pulling things off his shelves for the Christmas Express. They're all unsung heroes. Nobody asks for any credit or recognition. The businesses you think don't have a heart give quietly.*

Even businesses that you might not think would be a perfect fit found a way to help, like the Pilot House restaurant. For fourteen seasons, locals had thoroughly enjoyed their annual Christmas open house happy hour. What started out as a modest party for the regulars had evolved over the past few years into a gala event, but many were far more touched when they learned that the party had been canceled one year so that all of the money usually spent on the party could be donated to Christmas Express. The decision, according to the manager, was directly related to the current economic recession the area was experiencing. As the Christmas season crept closer and party plans were formulated, the management and staff questioned if it was responsible to fund free alcohol and hors d'oeuvres when so many families had more pressing needs. "We felt that we could put the money to a better use than just throwing a party."

Annie placed donation boxes for Christmas Express around her entire area. One year Annie's living room was full of gifts donated through a box in the nave by her church family at Calvary Baptist, which was not a wealthy church. She recalled the day when she was gathering donations at the church and a fellow church member, Betty Robinson, a woman in her 80s who couldn't walk well, came down the path with a group of friends.

> There were five little ladies limping down the path with their walkers, all wearing Santa hats. I looked out and saw them coming in this absolute parade of love. They brought wonderful gifts.
>
> I usually wait until after Christmas to write my many thank-you notes, but after these women left I had to sit down and compose my letter to them the very next morning.
>
> Dear Betty, the "Mighty Mite" Society, and Our Dear Church Family at Calvary Baptist:

I take pen in hand with a heart filled with gratitude. It is because of you all, your generous and loving hearts, that Christmas Express was able to not only pull out of the station, but was loaded with boxcars full of thoughtful, beautiful presents.

I did not think that physically I would be able to undertake the large responsibility of Christmas Express this year. I am mostly housebound now and knew that I could not shop. Well, Christmas arrives softly on the wings of angels . . . and in this instance our Calvary family has been the angels, messengers of the Lord, telling these needy and deserving families that God does care about them, that they are not alone. Your greatest gift was not in a box or wrapped in a bow. It was the gift of Christian charity and love. For this I can never thank you all enough.

With your encouragement, I began a telephone campaign soliciting donations, getting press reporters to interview on the phone! One reporter even came to our home this morning at 8:00 a.m. to do a story!

One candle, one hope, one act of compassion is bringing light and joy into the shadow of poverty.

Glenn, my quiet Santa, joins with me in our heartfelt gratitude to all of you at Calvary Baptist Church. We wish for you to embrace the joy of this holiday, recognizing that our Lord is with us always in all ways!

Love,
Annie and Glenn

Newspapers were very instrumental in putting out the word about Christmas Express, and many heartwarming and informative stories and photos were written about the special cause. Occasionally one of the reporters would focus too much on Annie and her motivations, celebrating her as a kind of saint, and this made her very uncomfortable.

I was adamant that it wasn't my special cause and that I desired no special attention for my organizing efforts. One year I spent two mind-wrenching days writing an article titled "Miracles of Christmas Past" for the newspaper to thank the generous community for their help. These people were "Angels of Christmases Past" and I wrote vignettes about their special acts, which had hitherto gone unrecognized. But the effort went off the track when a self-serving reporter completely cannibalized my article and wrote the story about me. My message went completely unheeded. This is NOT ABOUT ME. It really, really upset me.

I couldn't do this without my husband, who gives me so much support. He's the one who does most of the legwork. I'm the heart but he's the beat. He's the reason I'm still hopping. Without Glenn there would be no Christmas Express. He does it very quietly, and no one knows what this man does.

In many of the newspaper interviews that she did, Annie talked about Glenn. She called him her unsung Santa. Over the years, Christmas Express became their

Christmas. Whatever they had in donations, they would add to with their own donations.

> I don't think Glenn has ever gotten the socks or shirts and gloves I've bought for him because at the last minute I find out about a teenage boy who could use the gift. We try not to get each other presents until two days before Christmas.
>
> One Christmas Glenn gave me a wrapped box with a handmade card. The card had a bear on the front with the words "A Christmas wish just for Annie." Inside it read, "This little bear just looked so cute that right away I knew he had to be the one to bring this Christmas wish to you!" Then it continued, "Hi Annie, I had a little accident in the shop. Glenn accidentally chopped my arm off. Now I need a gentle home, NOT SOME LITTLE KID, so please don't give me away. As a one-armed bear, I'll hug back the best I can." In reality, the arm had been successfully replaced into the little bear's body, but Glenn was trying to get me to actually keep one of his gifts.

Donation boxes for Christmas Express did not only appear in places you would expect to see them like churches or libraries. They also popped up in restaurants, stores, and locations for sporting events. In addition to donation boxes, Annie would also use any reasonable means of attracting attention to her cause. One method that worked was to use one or more pets from her and Glenn's menagerie to draw curious onlookers so that Annie could tell them about Christmas Express.

Glenn and I caused some excitement at the Court House branch of Sturdy Savings Bank this year, with both of us attired in festive red-and-white Santa hats. Patrons, busily banking for their holiday shopping, were curious about the little creature that I was holding. It was Splice, our ferret. The branch manager, forewarned of the special arrival, got her turn to also wear a Santa hat as she held Splice. Our frisky ferret, puzzled about being the center of attention, didn't seem overly anxious to oblige as I placed a tiny elf's hat on him. Laughter abounded as Splice wiggled in the arms of the manager when I tried to right the wee hat atop Splice's head for a photo. Willing customers happily contributed that day to a large collection box that we had placed in the bank, inviting donations.

The ferret may have caused a little ruckus, but it was nothing compared to the scene at Steve's New Jersey Nature animal center later that week. There I posed with five huge Sulcata tortoises sporting antlers, their leader with a bright red ball for a nose. Those hefty African tortoises were indifferent to their role as reindeer replacements for a photo opportunity. They graciously bore their temporary brown pipe cleaner antlers that Steve, who owned the turtles, and I had taped to their shells. "Turtles can fly, snow in July. Anything is possible if you believe," I told the local reporter as I donned a red-and-white Santa hat for a picture and knelt behind a little wagon filled with toys in the backyard of Steve's home, where he has his reptile animal center. Of course behind the scenes it wasn't all that simple . . . .

Steve and I spent a hysterical half hour posing five tortoises. Dasher kept dashing off to the left while Dancer danced to the right. Their reins of red velvet ribbon kept falling off while Steve was trying to attach them to a toy-laden wagon. The photographer clicked away trying to bring order to the crazy Christmas scene unfolding before his rather incredulous eyes. Steve was a trooper, gathering the "reindeer" and keeping them in line while I ducked behind the sleigh, smiling away with my Santa hat at a drunken angle, all the while breathlessly giving copy to the reporter!

As the years went by, Christmas Express grew and so did Annie's health problems. Annie's bulldog efforts to have a bigger and better Christmas Express every year always landed her in bed for the next several weeks following the holidays.

During the Christmas Express season of 1998, Annie broke her foot, had one eye swollen shut, lost twenty-two pounds, and became anemic but did not want to let the kids and families down. Even though her mind was fogged by pain-killing narcotics (trying to counteract the severe flare-ups of her condition), she knew the list of people in need was long and it broke her heart.

After she survived that year, Annie started looking for that special person to whom she could pass the candle, someone who felt the need of children and their families and had the desire to carry on with what she had started and given so much of her life to. She gave a newspaper interview in which she pleaded for a new director:

> Last year it was too close, and it was scary, so I promised Glenn I would give up Christmas Express. I'm not trying to be dramatic, but I want people to understand that this really was a gut-wrenching decision. The stamina is gone. I'm depending too much on morphine. I don't want to get into it and then let the kids down. They're too important to me. I may be able to start it, but I don't have the momentum to keep it going. That's what made me decide that it's time to turn it over.
>
> Christmas Express is about hope. It's about the Christmas miracles that happen every year. What I'm pleading for is that the spirit, the light, and the love that is Christmas Express not be extinguished. I could not bear it if it was. If someone doesn't step in, there will be people who don't get presents or even food. I'm asking for one person or several to fill my shoes. All the merchants are very forthcoming, but they have to be approached in person, something I just can't do anymore. I consider Christmas Express an ongoing miracle and have faith that it will not stop when I hand over the reins to a new director.

Well, Annie got her miracle. A twenty-three-year-old substitute teacher, whose parents Annie had known for years, stepped in with fresh enthusiasm and energy. Annie officially passed her "I believe in Santa" hat to Amy Martin in an emotional little ceremony at the cabin along with all of the record books that would be so instrumental in the future success of Annie's cherished organization, which had helped so many families over the past sixteen years.

In the newspaper article featuring the passing of the torch, Amy said, "Annie has been a role model for me since I can remember. She is an amazing woman who has helped a lot of children through the years with the support of her husband, Glenn. I only hope that I can continue to do what she has done so successfully in the past."

With Annie's instruction and inspiration, Christmas Express didn't miss a beat under the direction of its new leader. With health and vitality, Amy took on Christmas Express and was able to not only keep it going but kept it growing.

As a tribute to Annie and her extraordinary dedication and accomplishments founding and running the Christmas Express, Annie was honored by having a day in New Jersey named after her. Middle Township Mayor Michael J. Voll read the township recognition and proclamation from Governor Jim Florio in a ceremony decreeing that, henceforth, January 16 would always be known as Anne Stites Appreciation Day.

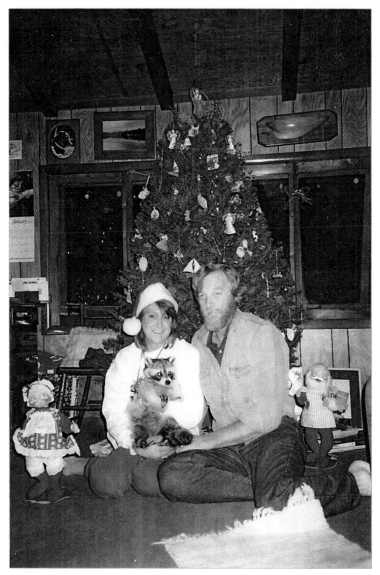

Christmas at Nature's Way

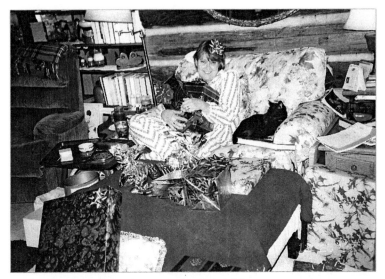

Annie loved Christmas with the heart of a child

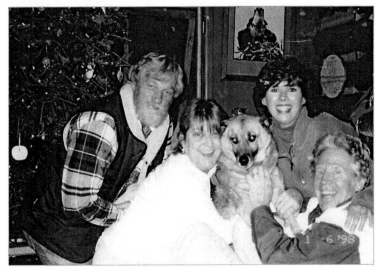

Gail and Ray visiting at Christmastime

CHAPTER EIGHT

Our Salvation

ONE DAY ANNIE SAID, "We live at the shore; we should have a boat." This sounded like an interesting idea to Glenn, and he was excited about the possibility. The next step was to decide what kind of a boat they should get. Glenn remembered a story about a man with serious osteoporosis who went out on the ocean for a ride in a powerboat. The continuous pounding that his body took every time the boat hit a wave caused him a great deal of pain, and he ended up in the hospital three inches shorter.

Given Annie's health, the option of a powerboat was quickly eliminated. Sailing was appealing to both of them as a sport that would allow them to be more at one with the sea. Glenn had heard about a sailing school in Annapolis, and they eagerly signed up and took the classes that began in the fall. Classes were held on shore in the morning and moved to one of several twenty-six-foot Rainbow boats for "hands on" lessons in the afternoon. Couples were split up and not allowed to be together on the same boat, the theory being that they would be more attentive and learn more if they were separated from their partner. Classes were small, with only five or six students aboard each boat.

Because it was the end of the sailing season, they would have to wait until spring for classes to continue. Over the winter Glenn read every book about sailing he could get his hands on. Early the following spring, before classes started up again, Glenn heard of someone who was selling his thirty-one-foot double-ended Norwegian sloop named *Freyja*, which means goddess of the sea. The King of Norway's boat was also named *Freyja*. Annie and Glenn were never ones to sit on their enthusiasm, so they bought the boat before they had even completed their classes!

Freyja was a Knud Reimers design, classified as a Fortuna Class racing sloop. It had a wooden hull and spar but was "dismasted" in a race off of Boston in the late 1950s—meaning that it could no longer compete professionally. It was rerigged as a masthead sloop with an aluminum spar and boom.

Now that they were officially boat owners, Glenn and Annie were eager to resume their classes that spring. Morning lessons were spent on the boat because they covered working the engine, systems, plumbing, refrigeration, and the necessary mechanics. The afternoon was the fun part where they would actually sail and apply all of the lessons that they had been learning. The captain would come aboard in the morning and get off at night, and the rest of the crew, made up of students, slept aboard. By this time Annie and Glenn were allowed on the same boat together!

After several weekends of sailing lessons, plans were made for their first solo cruise on the Chesapeake Bay. After making a well-thought-out list, they loaded up *Freyja* with supplies and pulled anchor.

That first day they raised their sails and made their way up the Cape May channel to the Delaware Bay and then sailed into the C&D (Chesapeake and Delaware) channel that would lead them to the Chesapeake Bay. It is against the law for boats to "sail" in the channels, so they lowered their sails and motored along at *Freyja's* top speed of five knots.

Ten hours after they had entered the channel and they had gone forty-eight miles, suddenly there was a wind shift and the current was now going against them. A fast current can be strong enough to create a wake around pilings of almost a foot high. Their speed slowed to barely moving. They could see people walking along the shore who were making better time than they were. At times their speed was five knots while the speed of the current was six knots and they were actually losing ground with twenty more miles to go before reaching the end of the channel. And then, hours later, while still battling the current and still with ten miles to go, they ran out of gas.

Glenn quickly raised the sails so we had steerage with the current, keeping us away from the rocks. I "calmly" called the Coast Guard. "Whiskey Roger Tango 6626, calling C.G." It sounded so nautical.

"Sailing vessel, Freyja, has run out of fuel in the center of the shipping lane." An answer came back that help was on the way within fifteen minutes. Andrea M., a tugboat out of Norfolk, Virginia, was coming to our rescue.

The tug's job and purpose is to tow major cargo ships through the channel. Cargo ships don't have the fine movement control it takes to navigate through the channel by themselves. It can take ten miles for these big ships to be able to stop. A C&D captain, who knows every inch of the bottom, goes aboard the ship and safely navigates it through the channel with help from the tugboat.

Within a few minutes, the tug pulled up alongside Freyja and passed a rope to Glenn. By law, the rope has to come only from the tugboat. Designed for towing large ships, the rope passed to Glenn was a two-and-a-half-inch maritime rope, making it very heavy and difficult to handle. Glenn then had to figure out how and where to secure it to our sailboat. After accomplishing that, Freyja was tied up tightly alongside the tugboat, sort of like a pontoon. Tire bumpers along the edge of the tug protected Freyja from damage. It was a bit nerve-wracking to be tied to the tug to our port side while moving at six knots. The scariest part came when they pushed us sideways into the dock at Schaeffer's, a fueling station and restaurant in the marina.

An audience had assembled on the dock. The dock boy dropped the bowline twice and the tug had to quickly reverse the engines. I had visions of one large matchstick where Freyja used to be. The dink folded completely in half. Glenn held on to the tiller for dear life. He was sure that the rudder was going to snap. I was on the bow throwing lines, trying to put bumpers on, plus release the tug line. All I could see was Lovie's legs flying up trying to balance himself. Panic set in.

The tug finally released us amid great cheers and horn blowing. They couldn't release the bowline, so they threw the entire 150 feet of one-and-a-half-inch dock line on Freyja. It was enormous. Schaeffer's hadn't seen so much excitement in years. People kept coming out of the restaurant to comment on the goings on. Glenn reveled in the well-deserved compliments about how beautiful Freyja is.

It was 10:00 p.m. before we were settled and headed to Rib and Chicken for much needed and delicious Planter's Punch. We took the hot ribs and chicken aboard to eat.

How lucky we are that all is okay. We turned in around 12:00 p.m. exhausted mentally and physically. Ah, the panic and peacefulness of sailing.

And so a trip to the Chesapeake that should have taken ten hours ended up taking twenty-two hours and included some unexpected adventure. The next day was Annie's birthday.

They were up at daybreak, the water was still, and just the sound of birds could be heard as they glided into the Chesapeake in the early morning hours. This was the first of many cruises that they would take to what became their favorite place, the Chesapeake Bay. Sailing provided Annie and Glenn with a glorious feeling; once they untied those lines from the dock and headed off into the bay, it was like they were untying shackles that bound them to the land. Financial worries, vocational worries, and of course health worries began to release their hold as soon as the breeze hit their faces. Several years later, and after becoming seasoned sailors on the Chesapeake Bay, Annie wrote:

> *What a joy to see a sunrise as my first glance of the day. I was up by 6:00 a.m. and put on coffee. Got tea and sodas ready for our journey to Annapolis. Yes, we are crossing the bay, a five-hour sail . . . . Captain Hippie is now explaining his desire to be on the "open sea," i.e., the Chesapeake. He has had enough of putting down creeks for a while.*
>
> *I am trying not to take pain meds. Usually I wake up in pain; it is my first sensation of the day, same old place, lower left quadrant. The pain itself doesn't bother me. Mr. P and I have been well acquainted for most of my life. I'm anxious, maybe a bit discouraged too, because I want so much just to feel well and have some energy. I refuse to give in to the desire to lie down a lot. I make myself go one more step, then one more until I'm distracted and not pain-centered. I brought a book along on pain control. It is difficult to really face the future*

of chronic pain, but I will not be defeated by it or let "it" control my life. I am learning visualization techniques and storing up tranquil images of our sojourn because I know that I can't keep taking a pill. I have been on constant pain meds for two years now and worry about the lasting effects.

We are both thoroughly enjoying the relaxed camaraderie of the marina fold. Everyone is so pleasant, and there is quite a cast of characters among these liveaboards.

Last night Debbie, our neighbor on Moon Dance, came aboard wanting to know about courses needed to become a teacher. Poor kid had a perfectly horrendous experience in school being labeled "learning disabled" and subsequently was mishandled by a line of inept teachers. She wants to be able to help kids like herself. We had a lively discussion about the many faceted realms of the teaching profession, i.e., administrative crap, political tangles, rigid curriculum code, lousy pay, etc. Of course all was said with a bit of wistfulness on my part. I am still unable to really accept that I'll never teach again. The hopeful thought remains, maybe next year. I am still trying to come to grips with it all. It has been one of the toughest decisions of my life. I know now that the risks far outweigh the benefits of gainful employment.

It makes me feel useless though, and I'm in limbo. I haven't been really strong enough to even commit to volunteer work. It's like a roller coaster, fine one day and pain the next.

I know God has a divine plan for my life, and I must be patient. Sometimes though, I really feel my life is over in the sense of goals that I have always had for myself. I know that sounds pessimistic and harsh but when I'm home alone in the morning after Glenn has left, I stare out the window and think, What am I going to do with myself? *I ease my way into a solitary day with a few phone calls and puttering through some domestic chores, which I still abhor. Just because I have boobs doesn't mean I am domestic Doris!*

I have plans to become involved with AAUW (American Association of University Women, an equality advocacy organization) and to better organize Christmas Express this year. I am also hatching an idea to take critters to nursing homes. I know there are many, many good and useful ways to spend my newfound boredom. The catch is I only have a few strong hours a day. Should I get a part-time job under the table that pays?

I cannot write anymore of the negative crap. I know I have a bounty of blessings, number one being my precious husband. This page, which bemoans my fate, is not an all-prevailing feeling with me. I'm just uncertain and a bit anxious about our future security. It is so very frustrating not to be able to contribute while watching our resources drain.

Enough, Anne. The Lord will provide. Glenn has always gotten us through. He is so talented. I am always so proud of him. I know we will never be rich, but if love were money we are already wealthy. I remember Glenn once saying with a wry smile, "We have a lot of wealth; we just can't spend it."

Just glanced back at Glenn who is back from his shower. His "redneck" tan is finally being filled in. He was pretty funny looking with his red neck and arms but white chest and legs. His legs are slowly getting tan and the shirt mark is almost gone. His broad, strong back is a stunning, sexy bronze. I may be feeling horny, but it's too damn hot to do much about it!

He looks like a sailing sultan perched on fluffy pillows, with the canapé overhead providing shade. The picture is completed by his sailing smile. His fingers need only to barely touch the wheel because Freyja has great tracking.

When it was finally time to "put in," the wind was a good fifteen knots with waves five to six feet and about eight dip 'n dive feet apart. We were soaked and salty, but happy just to be on the sea.

But oh, me and my Christopher Columbus ideas! After a glorious day with a cool, sunny sail, close haul for about an hour before the wind died, we entered Magothy. There was no problem entering but Broad Creek was another story. We ran aground once, twice, three, yes, four times! According to the chart, it should have been nine to fourteen feet deep all the way down. Ho, ho, the last time aground was a riot. "Ol' Captain Glenn" was a bit ticked off to put it mildly. His face was radiating sort of a red/

blue hue and his voice was down at least six octaves, definitely not a sign of joy. He jumped in the dinghy, switched on the motor, and thank heavens it started or I think it would have been taken apart bolt by bolt and tossed to the crabs. He then proceeded to unceremoniously ram Freyja on the port, then zoom around to starboard and ram again. I didn't dare open my mouth, but he really did look a sight with a dirty white sailing hat jammed on his head and a cigarette between battle-clenched teeth, but it worked. Freyja nosed off and we headed out of Broad Creek without a backward glance, off to Cattail Creek about three miles up.

We ended up in a nice cove to starboard with the cockpit facing a small stretch of woods and cul-de-sac. I do believe we are getting the hang of it! We arrived in St. Michaels at about 5:00 p.m. and anchored in a neat cove to starboard of the main harbor.

Glenn really scraped his hand on the anchor chain. There was blood all over the place! While we recouped in the cockpit, we were greeted by two hens and fourteen darling, wee baby mallards, oh, so precious. We fed them bread. Then two swans and four juveniles still with down swam over. Now I understand the story of The Ugly Duckling. *Heavens, they were a motley-looking bunch, gray with tufts of down all over, with a feather or two peeking out in incongruous places. Of course, knowing us, they ended up with all the bread we had.*

Later in the day we rowed into the Crab House for a sumptuous feast. We had a whole lobster, oysters, and king crab. Glenn started off ordering a banana daiquiri. He got giddy on three and kept saying, "This is nice, think I'll have another."

A breathtaking full moon came into view as we dined. We giggled and laughed as we rowed back to Freyja in the moon-drenched waters. Back on Freyja we "christened" the cockpit just as a launch with a spotlight came by. Glenn's face was an array of colors. What a riot!

Glenn was Annie's hero in many ways and her rock, not only through her physical travails but as her life partner. She felt safe with Glenn as a competent and calm person when things got rough. Together they would embrace the often extreme weather conditions found in the sailing life with exuberance and a little bit of fear mingled with delight at the spectacular show they happened to be witnessing. Annie would sit on the bridge deck with the cold rain and wind slapping her face, but by hugging Glenn she could feel his warmth through his jacket and feel safe and protected.

During one particular storm though, Glenn was off at work, and even though *Freyja* was in their boat slip, Annie had quite the time of it by herself:

The bay is churning, tossing wildly; fifty to fifty-five knot gusts drive the waves that are cascading over the bulkhead and slamming into the companionway. The wind is literally howling. Freyja is rocking and straining at her lines. I have never been aboard during such turbulence. My heart won't stop pounding; it skips a beat with each crash of the sea on the coach house. The canvas is flapping wildly, and I'm waiting for the covers to snap at any second.

There is such fury and turmoil, whereas yesterday the bay was tranquil and beckoning. Gads, things are really wailing. Nine tons of boat is heeling 15 percent.

Glenn was off early this morning to work, but I wish he were here so I could continually ask, "Sure we are okay?" though it feels and sounds like we are going to blast apart. Oh God, there was just a great flash of light as the canvas flew off!

The hull is pounding and thumping in the slip. Rocking crazily, I keep realizing that I am gritting my teeth and have to talk aloud to stop from clenching them. I tried to take a few pictures, so I raised the camera, wrapped in a baggie, out of the hatch just as a wave broke over the bulkhead and caught me full on. I was drenched in one second.

I'm unable to leave Freyja alone without help. I wouldn't be able to even get over the stern rail to the bulkhead much less walk down the bulkhead. The force of the wind and spray would be too much.

Oh where is Glenn!? Every thump in the cockpit causes me to look hopefully for his dripping wet countenance. I cannot believe that I am actually getting seasick in the slip! Freyja is shuddering and yanking crazily. My only fear is that there will be damage. Words are inadequate to describe this heart-thumping, adrenaline-pumping storm.

Classical music is playing, hoping to soothe my rather rattled nerves. Hot tea is on the table, and our cat Mizzen, is curled up under the lamp. Who Me, Mizzen's son, is forward on the V-berth shelf fast asleep, how I'll never know. I even tried to close my eyes to absorb some Beethoven. That lasted one second.

Freyja is pouncing from beneath every possible line, and every shackle or stay is rattling wildly. The cover canvas is giving me heart failure with every blast of wind. I'm tempted to reach out from the port and cut the poor tortured thing loose.

I still marvel over the sheer force and anger of the turbulent sea. It was smooth as satin yesterday and a churning, white foaming Goliath today. How would I react if we were actually on the sea during this kind of madness? After wetting my pants, I really don't think I could make it through this kind of storm. That is a hard reality to face. We have been such fair weather sailors.

You really have to have faith in your vessel, and I do on Freyja. The cockpit floorboards were flooded. Frantically I moved the heater, put the wet kitty litter on the counter, and opened the engine door. The bilge was filling fast. There was ten minutes of sheer panic as I furtively searched for the manual bilge pump, but pump to where?

Yikes, Mike from a neighboring boat just leaped aboard and to be heard over the howling wind, yelled, "I'll be back in fifteen minutes." Not knowing what the hell to do, I scrambled forward and repacked the exit duffle with dry clothes for us, cat chow, makeup, and a hair dryer. I stuffed money in my jacket along with my pills and emptied the other duffle bag to toss cats in if we had to leave fast. I felt absolutely helpless.

Stopping back aboard, Mike told me that the scuppers had been cleared and Freyja wasn't going to sink. I thanked him for that bit of reassurance. I have been staring out the companionway. Waves are breaking into the cockpit. I've never seen the bay so wild with such force and majestic power of nature; it is humbling to say the least.

Gotta admit, Hippie, my nerves are beginning to get frazzled. And I'm not alone! Poor Who Me is wide-eyed and rather freaked. I've had him on my lap to calm him but I'm rocking too. I put him in the boat bag and covered him with a shirt, and now with one golden watchful eye, he is peering out at me.

I sure am missing you, Captain, and would feel a lot better if you were sitting across from me reassuringly saying, "Everything is okay."

Glenn got back to the boat in the late afternoon as the storm was dying down, and Annie was overjoyed to see him. It is common for sailors such as Mike to take care of each other, provided they know where to find you!

Annie and Glenn were never hard to find. They attracted a lot of attention not only with their fun-loving ways, but because of the animal menagerie they often brought with them when they came to the Chesapeake to sail. Boaters frequently bring their dogs aboard, but leave it to Annie and Glenn to also bring cats, ferrets, and even raccoons!

> *Critter crew is aboard. Mizzen and Who Me are old sea salts. Splice the ferret is experiencing his first sail and is into, on top of, and burrowing under everything. Tippy is aboard too. We would never leave him at home. He is so good on the boat and absolutely loses it when we leave him. Tippy is sporting his summer buzz cut, checkered with nearly bald patches where the clipper snagged. Glenn said I should be reported for animal abuse. Tippy is giving me the sad doe eyes. What have you done to me?*
>
> *Unbelievably we upped hook at 7:30 a.m. No time to go for "shore leave" for Tippy. Now it is 6:30 p.m. and Tippy has not gone to the bathroom yet. I took him forward to the green Astroturf on the bow and demonstrated. I kept lifting his leg saying, "It's okay, go! Go!" Glenn was cracking up, and Tippy was eyeing me like I was insane. I cannot understand how he is holding it in. I swear his eyes are bulging.*
>
> *The gang at the marina went bonkers over our baby raccoon, Noah, each holding him and taking pictures. I got a kick out of the burly marine workers absolutely melting when cradling Noah in their*

roughened work hands. Their serious, suntanned
faces were softened with smiles as they held Noah.
The biggest one of all extended a tentative finger to
Noah's mouth and said, "Hey, look, he's holding my
finger." He was absolutely thrilled and didn't want
to release him.

Noah had come into Annie and Glenn's life after their beloved Pepper passed. Pepper had become quite a sailor spending months aboard *Freyja* with Annie and Glenn. He adapted well to the boat and enjoyed the freedom of the vessel.

In the wild a raccoon is lucky to live eight to ten years, but in the comfort and safety of their home, Pepper lived happily for nineteen years.

When Annie and Glenn were living on the boat in Annapolis, after going out to dinner one evening they came back to the boat and played with Pepper for a while before going to bed. The next morning Glenn got up at 5:00 a.m. to go to work. He was having his morning coffee, and Pepper came up to him and put his arms out to be lifted up into Glenn's arms as he so often did. A moment later his body went limp. He died peacefully in Glenn's arms.

Taking care of a raccoon for me is one of the most
special experiences I could ever imagine in life. This
past Wednesday in the late afternoon I made a call
to Jody at Cape Vet inquiring about taking care of
baby squirrels that were orphaned in last week's

squall . . . . It turned into something joyous and truly amazing!

When she told me about an orphaned, injured raccoon, my stomach did a flip-flop in anticipation. I gulped with tears filling my eyes. "Jody, oh Jody, do you think we could care for him? Oh jeez, you know how much we have longed for a baby since Pepper died." Jody told me that Bill was caring for him at the animal rehab. It was too late to call him today, damn. I was afraid to hope too much. Silently, I was pleading with the angels of fate that they would allow us to care for this precious, injured baby.

The next morning I called Bill and with my heart in my mouth I asked about the baby raccoon. The words I heard made my whole world come crashing down, and with tears streaming down my face I said, "Sure, I understand, of course your wife is attached to the baby. Please let me know if there is anything I can do to help." I got off of the phone, and with all that I had hoped for having just been shattered, I had a good cry.

I got back to Jody on Friday to find out what supplies I should get for the baby squirrels. Skipping my question, she quickly asked, "Didn't Bill call you?"

Sensing something was up by the urgency in her voice, I held my breath and simply answered, "No."

Jody continued, "Annie, after an 'all-nighter' with the baby raccoon, bunnies, and birds, Bill's wife realized what a good home the baby raccoon would have with you and said you could have him."

Tears of disbelief followed a war whoop of sheer joy. Our dream was coming true. "Glenn, GLENN, we can have the baby," I shouted.

Ah, Noah, our prayers for a baby raccoon have been answered. It was so unexpected. I never even knew that raccoons had litters as late as August.

A violent thunderstorm three weeks ago toppled this little kit from his tree trunk nest. He was discovered but left on the ground for twelve hours before anyone took him for help, hoping the mother would reclaim her baby. But survival of the fittest is nature's iron clad rule and it was not to be broken.

Unable to lift his head and obviously injured with a concussion, it is possible that he will have permanent brain damage as well as the loss of his left eye. An infected and festering wound on his back is also of concern. Mama had left him to the elements and certain death.

Trembling with anticipation I raced to the rehab to meet and take home our new baby and was tripping on Bill's heels as we wound our way through the clinic to the back treatment room. Bill brought forth this four-inch, fuzzyheaded baby so young that his ears were still curled forward. His nose was blunt and he had a wide nursing mouth. His tiny little paws touched Bill's nose as Bill nuzzled him and said, "Good-bye, little fella, you have a new mommy now."

As tears were rolling unheeded down my face, I reached tentatively, eagerly for this wee, sick orphan, still not quite believing our good fortune.

Memories of Pepper as a baby came flooding forth. Pepper was our treasured pet, our child, for nearly two decades. The void left by his death still aches. So often, especially at night when we are laying on our pillows, I see his face, the sensation of his paws gently searching my face and head, and feel his strong warm furry body as we would hug and cuddle. So many times coming up those steps, I still see him in our bed, eager face, ready to play or say hello. His bright ink-black eyes vibrant and mischievous, fuzzy soft ears bent forward in anticipation, and front paws working to remove the covers that surround him. Then there was that singular two-step and a hop as he would rush to the edge of the bed and grab hold of my waiting arms. I cry now remembering him, but now is the time for happiness again . . . .

This is not to say that caring for an injured baby raccoon was easy, especially aboard a sailboat! It was daily, hourly work to heal Noah's wounds, nourish him, help him with his coordination, and encourage him to first sit upright and then to crawl.

Noah's appetite has increased markedly as he grows. The feeding schedule is a bit wearing but at least not every hour or so. With a full belly, I lull him to sleep on my chest as his velvet paws gently caress and explore my face. He is wide-eyed when he finds my mouth and the pace of his moving fingers increases as he pries open my lips. "Wow, what's that, teeth? Smooth with all those neat cracks between them."

Reluctantly with a sigh he resigns himself to sleep, uttering little grunts as he settles his head sideways and soon is fast asleep. Often I will hum knowing it feels like his mother's purring. He definitely responds and is calm.

Noah is always the first one up in the morning, chuckling quietly at first then building in intensity and crescendo until he feels a warm hand lifting his furry being. Oh, that face, that curious, bright-eyed face! With velvet paws all working at once reaching toward you, his little countenance could melt granite with one look and one soft touch.

One morning after my morning prep of getting the coffee on, I went back to fetch Noah. He wasn't there! He had pushed aside the quilt and climbed out of his pen over the stacked pillows. I was frantic when I couldn't find him under the covers. My worst fear was realized as I spotted his furry head by the mast. He had fallen three feet to the hard cabin floor. My heart was in my throat, and a wave of sheer panic gripped me as I reached for him. His little upturned trusting face raised to my voice, paws moving. Oh God, is he hurt? I cannot believe my stupidity, but I couldn't foresee his strength and tenacity. He had never climbed out of his pen before. I rushed topsides with him and put him on a boat cushion to check mobility. He seemed to be unaffected, the hardheaded little bugger.

I am sitting in an idyllic spot now as I write about this, a small spit of beach on a marsh-tipped jut of land across from Freyja, leaning against a log with the water lapping gently at my feet. Noah is asleep in his boat bag next to me. Tippy is curled up in the sand watching for Glenn who went back to Freyja to run the reefer and futz for a while. When we beached the dinghy this morning, Glenn gave it a good wash down and then we took Noah for his first walk in the soft trodden marsh grass. He stood on all fours and then walked his very first steps! Oh no, here comes trouble! How to coon proof Freyja is going to be a challenge for our October cruise.

A new schedule is emerging. Early morning is the time for gentle self-play in the boat bag for an hour or so with the kitten toys that Glenn got for him, his favorite being the plastic ball with a bell that has lots of holes for prying fingertips. When he gets bored, he climbs out of the boat bag and begins tentatively exploring the floor. Oh boy, watch out. He gets two ounces of formula around 11:00 a.m. and is then rocked to sleep. Once soundly asleep, he is put into his "banky," a knit watch cap, and placed ever so carefully in his pen so as to not wake him.

Noah is a time-consuming, sleep-stealing, curious, adorable, worrisome little furry bundle of joy, and we love having him aboard with us.

The truth was, Annie and Glenn couldn't resist any animal that needed help and appeared to have no other way of receiving that help. One day while out doing last-minute errands, Annie and Glenn found an abandoned kitten wandering around in a parking lot. The very next day, Annie and Glenn were going to be leaving for a two-month sailing odyssey on the Chesapeake.

The timing wasn't great for adopting another animal, but they certainly couldn't just ignore this helpless baby. From the condition she was in, they knew she would never make it on her own, so they squeezed into their already busy schedule an extended visit to the vet. After more than an hour, and a couple of hundred dollars later, they left the vet's office trying to think of a name for their new kitten.

They boarded *Freyja* the next morning with the little cat. She adapted to the boat so well that she was given the name Mizzen, the name of a sailboat mast. It was two months before she again stepped paw on land.

A year later Mizzen gave birth to a litter of kittens and homes were found for all of them but one, who they couldn't resist keeping. This little guy had a knack for knocking over just about everything in his way. He would then look at you with an expression on his face that asked, who me? And so "Who Me" became his name.

When Annie and Glenn were living aboard *Freyja*, Mizzen and Who Me would sometimes get off the boat at night to prowl the docks. One night Who Me was insistent about waking Annie and Glenn who were both sound asleep. He jumped on Glenn's chest meowing incessantly and then went to Annie to wake her as well. At first their reaction was to brush this annoying cat off of them, but he was relentless in his determination to wake them. He rubbed their heads, pushing and meowing, his eyes wide like yellow saucers.

Once he succeeded in waking them, he jumped off of the berth, ran a few feet, stopped, and turned around to see if they were following. He repeated this procedure several times, which was unusual behavior for him, and that's when they finally realized that he was on a mission. Annie and Glenn shot out of the berth knowing instinctively that something was wrong. They quickly looked around for Mizzen and as half-expected, there was no sign of her. Suddenly they realized what Who Me was trying to tell them.

It was the middle of winter, raining and cold. They hurriedly fumbled into their foul-weather gear and with flashlights in hand made a frantic search of the water around the boat, fear and tears flowing with each passing minute. "Mizzen, Mizzzeeen . . ." Their voices were lost in the wind. Panic set in, and they couldn't ignore that dreadful feeling that comes when someone you love is missing.

Who Me was their only hope of finding her, so when he jumped off the boat and started down the dock Annie and Glenn were close behind. They ran down the bulkhead, spotlighting the timbers underneath. "Oh Glenn, oh no . . . no . . ." Annie was looking but unseeing through a haze of tears. She was frantic but trying to calm herself so as not to lose control.

The rain was freezing cold, but their only concern was for Mizzen, who could be in trouble out there somewhere, and the weather conditions were making it worse. How long had she been gone? Why hadn't she returned to the boat with Who Me? Annie prayed that they would be able to find her. They just had to find her! As their frantic cries for Mizzen rang out in the marina, they saw boat lights starting to come on.

Suddenly Who Me stopped at a piling and started meowing and looking down at the water. In response a weak, plaintive wail was heard. Annie ran over and turned her light toward that beautiful sound and there she was, soaked, with ears like a bat, clinging fearfully to a piling just above the water's edge. Annie screamed for Glenn.

Mizzen was trapped. The bulkheads prevented her from being able to swim to shore and the new pilings with smooth plastic coverings were impossible to climb. Mizzen was clinging desperately to the piling, her little body half in the water with the tide rising.

By this time half the marina had been awakened by the ruckus. The boat owners, alarmed and curious, were gathering to see what the problem was and offering to help if possible.

The only way that Mizzen could be reached was for Glenn to balance like a tightrope walker on a rope that stretched from the dock down to a boat. There was a second, higher rope that he could hold onto for balance, and by traversing these ropes he was able to reach out and grab Mizzen with one hand and lift her up to Annie, who was kneeling on the dock reaching down for her.

Once Annie had Mizzen in her arms, a cheer went up from the concerned bystanders. Annie immediately wrapped the wet, terrified, and shivering cat in her sweatshirt. Annie and Glenn thanked their friends while apologizing for getting them up in the middle of the night and then hurried back to the boat to care for their traumatized little cat.

Mizzen was dried with a soft towel and then wrapped in a blanket and held against Annie's body until she was warm and had stopped shaking. Throughout this whole process, she was purring with gratitude.

Annie was still crying, but now with relief. Who Me had literally saved his mother's life. They gave him lots of love and praised him for being so smart. Annie almost squeezed the wind out of him, hugging and hugging. He was their little hero.

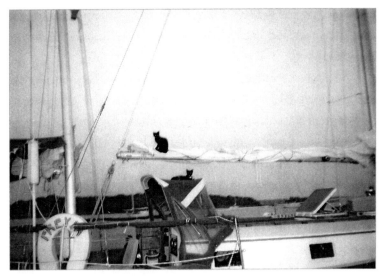

Cats Who Me and Missen sitting on the boom of *Freyja*

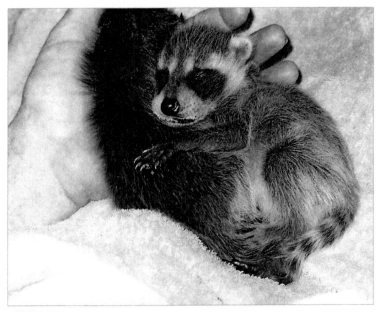

Infant Noah

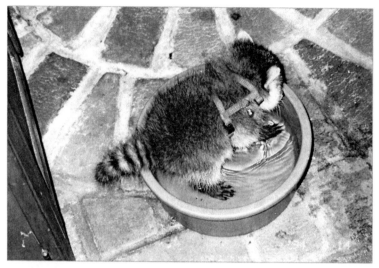

Baby Noah enjoys playing in water

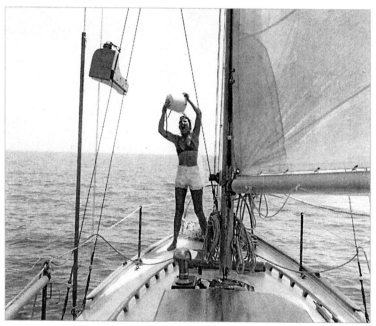

That's one way to cool off

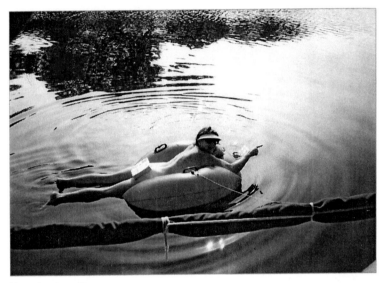

Have book, will cover

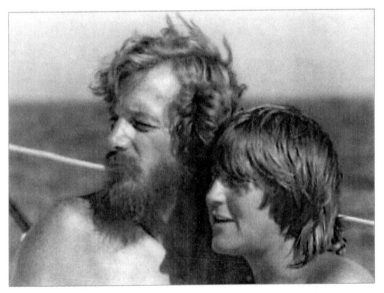

Together as one

CHAPTER NINE

This Renewed Life

The cats are racing all over the boat. Whoever wrote, "Fog crept in on little cat's feet" never stayed on a boat with cats! Thundering hooves on the coach house roof is always my morning wake-up call. The full moon has them really wired, darting in and out of ports and then racing down the deck, tails high and wild-eyed as they leap onto the dodger and smack whoever is up there, claiming triumphant king of the mountain.

Who Me is not about to stand for any impudence from young Blooper. He tackles her full on with a body slam onto the canvas. She spins around, ears flat, up on hind feet, bap, bap boxing style, and the chase is on. They thump to the deck and race to the bow. Blooper jumps into the forward hatch and *lands inches from Glenn's snoring head. He then stops to lick Mama Mizzen who waves a tolerant paw toward the brat, thwaping her pipe cleaner of a tail on the cabin floor.*

I remember being freaked over having our cats confined to a boat after the freedom of the cabin and woods. I had nightmares over the fear of them falling overboard, jumping onto other boats, or going off down the dock and getting lost on land. Oh, the worry but all for naught.

They took a while to adjust to noises, water, other cats, etc., but soon became part of the marina gang, up at night carousing about. Mizzen stayed aboard pretty much, lying on top of the dodger, keeping her eye, her good one, for she was blind in the other, out for Who Me until she saw him strutting back down the dock, tail high like he owned the place. Then she would get up to greet him.

One night I saw Who Me scamper down our dock with a buddy beside him. They came to Freyja, and Who Me hopped on board as if to say this is where I live. But as soon as his friend approached to jump aboard, Who Me chased him off with a "Hey, this is my boat, got it?"

The next night there was a whistling, howling, obstreperous wind, so I barely slept. Freyja was like a bucking bronco all night. I bounced out of the V-berth at 4:40 a.m., unable to stand it one more second. Poor Tippy at our heads was trying to come up with us while the cats were all huddled on the settee.

The sky is a stormy steel gray. White caps are in the anchorage with the wind blowing fifteen to twenty knots. No Baltimore today! We upped anchor as soon as Captain was alert enough after coffee to be able to function.

On this cold, wet day, we are off to Back Creek to seek respite from the howling and pounding. There were no other options for us with small craft warnings up and looking at the white caps and high seas. Our destination is one to two hours away, close enough. Gulp! Off we go after battening down everything below including the critters. Cats are all put in the V-berth, which is lined with blankets and pillows, and locked in by latching the opening head door. Our little ferret, Splice, was snug in her cozy little house under the V-berth. Tippy is topsides in the cockpit wearing a harness and we've donned our offshore suits.

Yow-eeee, what a breath-sucking, adrenaline-pumping, pants-wetting two hours! We pummeled our way through four-foot seas with twenty-knot winds on our nose all the way. Once out of protection of land, the games began. I braced myself against the gas box with one foot on the mizzen mast for balance.

Tippy was between my legs wearing his little red foul-weather jacket. His eyes were mournful but *trusting. Why are you doing this? he seemed to be saying. No answer there!*

Waves above the bow are crashing down on the forward deck with a flood from the sea, cascading down the decks to the cockpit. Rogue waves that intermittently come crashing onto a beam shower us with cold spray. It is a tumultuous, bow-slapping, bucking bronco ride! I find myself using all hitherto unknown muscles to hang on. Are we having fun yet?

Offshore suits are an absolute dry miracle. Pounding and chugging along, I look over Glenn's shoulder to waves cresting above him. Dear solid Freyja is bucking and crashing. The skyline of Annapolis is comforting, but there is still a ways to go.

Then crash—bang, the boom came loose. The pulley on the topping lift snapped from the pressure of the swing boom and fell onto the dodger and then slid off onto the winch, missing my head by inches.

Totally freaked now, I was shaking. Should we be doing this? Too late now. "We will be fine," I tell myself. Tippy is trying to crawl inside his jacket, poor pup.

As we neared Horn Point, we met with calmer water and limped on down to our cove in Back Creek, where we sipped hot coffee and checked on the critters, gingerly stepping around hurled Meow Mix. Wide-eyed Blooper was curled around Who Me. Mizzen, an old sea salt, was snug in the blankets purring, *What's all the fuss about?*

At times like this, Annie was really living. She loved excitement, and these thrills provided by nature satisfied the side of her that was a bit of a daredevil. Surviving the storms of the Chesapeake gave Annie and Glenn the confidence in their seamanship to attempt a lifelong dream of theirs: to sail the Caribbean seas, which they did three times. The first time, however, it seems that they were not as prepared as they thought they were. That adventure to the Caribbean was just a few months after they had finished only their first fall classes in Annapolis and had read a few books on sailing. At the time they thought they knew enough to try their hand at sailing their first boat.

That February they flew to Tortola in the Caribbean and chartered a twenty-two-foot Squibb sloop for the day. They sailed across the Sir Francis Drake Channel and soon realized that they didn't have a clue as to what they were doing. Evidently there is more to it than what you can learn in one weekend of classes and from reading a few books. Their destination was Peter Island. They had brought along some sailing books for reference, and the cruise became a "learn as you sail" kind of thing. They had some good laughs at their arrogant assumption that sailing could be so easy. Luckily they had open water in which to experiment, so no harm was done and a great deal was learned.

Through trial and error, they finally arrived at Peter Island. Glenn dropped anchor but couldn't figure out how to back up to tighten the slack, so he dove down and tied the anchor to a huge piece of corral.

With snorkeling gear they swam to the island that was about 200 yards away. As soon as they reached the beach, they were met by a beach guard who informed them that this was a protected beach and he couldn't allow them to come ashore. A bit disappointed, they swam back to the boat, had lunch, and sailed back to Tortola. The sail back was more successful than the trip to the island, but what could have been a six-hour cruise turned into an eight-hour sailing lesson.

With much more time and sailing experience under their belts, their second sailing adventure in the Caribbean was on a thirty-one-foot Bombay clipper named *Dancing Bear*. It was a lovely, peaceful, and fun vacation where they spent two weeks island hopping. Arriving at an island, they would drop anchor and dinghy in to a beach bar where they joined other sailing enthusiasts and everyone had a great time sharing boating stories. Some of the beach bars were exclusive to boaters because the only way to reach the beach was by boat. Beach bars were a fun place to come ashore and meet other sailors for a little camaraderie. One evening Annie and Glenn dinghied in to a beach bar and met a couple from Sweden. Conversation flowed easily and so did the drinks.

It was a friendly little circular bar surrounded by stools in the sand and protected by a palm roof. That night the bar was offering a buy one, get one free drink special and all that you could eat of the complimentary conch fritters that were being fried up right there. They had a great time drinking and laughing, and eating and drinking some more. It wasn't until they were making their way back to the dinghy that they realized how drunk they both were, drunk and horny. In their inebriated state, they hurried back to the boat as fast as they could, giggling the whole way. Less than gracefully they climbed the ladder, but didn't get much farther. Once topside the clothes started flying off, and their desire wasn't going to wait another minute. The closest place was the top of the cockpit and there, in the open air with probable witnesses, they made wild drunken love.

The third and longest sailing cruise was made possible with a bonus from their insurance company. Annie had a policy that paid fifty dollars a day for every day that she was in the hospital. This policy plays the odds, and Annie was one of the few who tipped the scales in her favor. They collected four thousand dollars and planned a month-long trip sailing in the Caribbean.

Summing up airfare, supplies for the boat, and extra spending money, four thousand wasn't enough to give them a full month of sailing, but if they shared the first two weeks with another couple they could swing it.

Glenn made reservations with a charter agency for a thirty-one-foot boat that would cost three thousand for a month. A few weeks later that company went belly up and was bought by another charter company who informed them that they didn't have a thirty-one-foot boat available. They did, however, have a thirty-five-foot boat, and they would let them have it for the same price as the thirty-one-foot boat.

Closing in on their vacation date, they again got a call from the agency this time telling them that the thirty-five-foot boat had just sunk. However, they had a forty-two-foot boat available, and they would honor the same price they had agreed on for the thirty-five-foot boat, which was the same price that they were originally going to pay for the thirty-one-foot boat.

So with this unlikely but extremely lucky chain of events, the originally chartered thirty-one-foot sloop turned into a forty-two-foot Morgan sailboat. Normally, the forty-two-foot upgraded boat would have given them one week of sailing for three thousand, but what they got was a month on the water for the same price.

Compared with the thirty-one-foot Sloop that was originally going to be their boat, the forty-two-foot Morgan Out Island Ketch with two masts and three sails was very luxurious. It was large enough to accommodate eight people, so for the first two weeks the four of them had a great time with so much space. The friends who sailed with them enjoyed scuba diving. They wanted to dive down to see the wreckage of the *Rome*, so Glenn pulled into an island near the site of the wreck. Glenn and Annie stayed on the boat while their friends dove to explore.

Within minutes after their friends had jumped overboard, a strong wind picked up. It wasn't raining but the sky was gray and the clouds were moving swiftly. A storm was coming from the other side of the island, and then with little warning there were sixty- to seventy-mile-an-hour winds.

Suddenly they were startled by a loud noise as the forward hatch, made of Plexiglas with a heavy teak frame, was ripped from its hinges and flew up over the mizzen mast thirty-five feet high and out to sea.

The entire storm lasted for about twenty minutes, and then it was over as fast as it had come. When their friends surfaced, they were all amazed that the divers had been completely unaware of any disturbance at all.

In parts of the Caribbean, there is what is referred to as the "Christmas winds." These unpredictable winds can be extremely strong and usually appear in November or December. The rest of the year is calm with gentle breezes that are called the "Trade winds."

Beef Island is a little island that got its name because the inhabitants raise cows. It has a small airport where sometimes a few cows have to be chased from the runway before an airplane can land, and this is where they dropped off the couple who had sailed with them for the first two weeks. Although Annie and Glenn had a great time with their friends, they both agreed that the last two weeks with just the two of them were the best.

It is a nice sail from Beef Island to Virgin Gorda. Glenn, Annie, and about fifteen other boats were making the same voyage. Suddenly it started to rain, and the wind came up blowing thirty-five miles per hour with stronger gusts. Winds of this velocity really test a sailor. All of the other boats arrived at their destination with quite a bit of damage. Sails were blown out, looking like shredded sheets hanging from the mast, and stays that hold up the mast were broken. Glenn and Annie's boat was the only one still intact, which gave them the satisfied feeling that they were seasoned and skillful sailors.

They felt bad for the others with damaged boats because they knew that their sailing vacation had just ended. There are a limited amount of boats to charter, and there are always more people who want to sail than there are available boats. Reservations are only safely made a year in advance.

Knowing that they would want to explore, Glenn took along a guidebook of the Caribbean and saw a place called Mary's Creek that looked interesting. The book showed no map, photographs, or drawings, just an explanation of how to get into Mary's Creek.

They motored into the entrance of the creek, which was one mile wide with no markers and was peppered with brain coral. The coral didn't move, so hitting one would put a big hole in the bottom of your boat. Making your way around them was like moving through a minefield. There could be as little as twenty feet between the many large pieces of brain coral, making it nearly impossible for the forty-two-foot boat to navigate around each one. Annie and Glenn felt like they were on the *African Queen*. The many groupings of coral lay underwater, and the only clue to their location was a small dark spot, which was only visible when you were about six feet away from any one of them.

Once past the entrance, the creek was well protected by land and about a block wide but extremely shallow and twisting.

Their plan to swim was deterred by the sight of sharks, so instead of swimming, they entertained themselves by tying string around pieces of chicken and dipping them into the water, enticing the sharks to come closer so they could have a better look. It was both exciting and a little scary to see these meat-eating sharks devour the chicken with one big snap of their jaws.

Unexpectedly, as one of the pieces of meat was being lowered to the water, a white bat with a twelve-inch wingspan swooped down, grabbed the piece of meat, and flew off through the skies, trailing a long piece of string behind him.

At the end of their vacation when they returned the boat to the charter company, the people couldn't believe that they had taken the boat into Mary's Creek and successfully navigated their way in and out of it. Familiar with the hazards they encountered, they were amazed and relieved that Glenn had brought the boat back undamaged.

Charter companies allow four to five days to make repairs on a boat before releasing it to another vacationer. The company was very much surprised and impressed to find that, especially after having been out for a month, there was no damage to repair except for the missing hatch cover that was now floating out in the ocean somewhere. With Glenn's skill and knowledge of boats, whenever something needed fixing, Glenn would just take care of it.

On the last night, the Christmas winds had died down and the rain was just a light sprinkle. A beach bar was at the top of the peninsula, and Annie and Glenn climbed up 200 feet to reach it. They enjoyed appetizers and drinks, and it was midnight before they came back down to the beach. There was still a light misting in the air, but the sky had cleared of clouds and there was a full moon. Enough light illuminated the sky to reveal a magnificent double rainbow. It was the kind of sight that stops you dead in your tracks with its awesome beauty. To make the moment even more magical, there was music drifting across the water from a boat in the harbor. A man was playing a guitar and singing in French the well-known and beloved hymn, "The Old Rugged Cross." They sat on the cool sand to suspend and absorb this ethereal moment and gaze at the rainbow that started from their boat and went up over an island and out into the ocean. At this moment and time in their lives, everything was perfect.

But as much as Annie and Glenn enjoyed their Caribbean vacations, they were always happy to be back home again on their beloved Chesapeake Bay.

We leapt out of the V-berth at 5:00 a.m., a half hour behind schedule, which we had carefully mapped out last night. Glenn and I were stretched out nude in the V-berth, chart in hand and tide books at the ready. It took a while to figure it all out. It's been a long time since we made a bay crossing.

What a glorious, cool morning it is as we get underway back on our "home" waters of the Chesapeake. The rosy predawn mist is like a bridal veil draping the shoreline; it's like sailing on a cloud. The fireball sun pops over the trees as we approach the Bay Bridge with ghostly silhouettes of big rigs crossing over. Steely glints of reflected sun were winking at us through the haze. We must have passed under this bridge hundreds of times over the years, and it still takes my breath away. It is a huge expanse, a marvel of man's ability to traverse nature's barriers. Cars and trucks, looking like Matchbox toys, are moving overhead, scurrying to their destinations. I went forward with Tippy to lie on the bow and look up as our mast passed under the whirring road overhead. A trick of perception gives the illusion of the mast tip nearly touching the bottom of the bridge.

I stand up in the cockpit giving my Miss America wave to buzzing traffic high over our heads. So many times as we drove cross the bridge, we gazed out of our car windows at the sailboats on the bay, longing to be there among them. Now here we are looking up with joy. We are here!

America is waking up and on the move.

Being on a boat in Annapolis Harbor is a spectacular place to be for the Fourth of July activities. Annie was a true patriot and loved the fireworks that celebrate the independence of our country. What was so much fun about Annie was that she was always ready and eager to enjoy any festivity to the fullest and in this case she was like a child seeing the fireworks for the first time.

It was a rousing, foot stompin', Sousa marching, God Bless America evening in the cockpit amid a gaggle of boats. The fireworks were loud and lovely, really breathtaking.

Before sunset, I donned my patriotic boxers and with a four-inch flag in hand, proceeded to march around the cockpit to the triumphant, soul-stirring cadence of Sousa marches, singing loudly and joyously to the "Battle Hymn of the Republic," "God

Bless America," and "My Country, 'Tis of Thee," all blaring forth from the cockpit speakers. Glenn with wads of toilet paper in his ears kept sinking lower and lower behind the coamings, trying in vain to disassociate himself from his screaming, patriotic, and utterly embarrassing wife.

As a small sailboat that was flying a huge American flag passed by, I put on "God Bless America." The sailors aboard saluted us and waved. Glenn was having apoplexy at this point.

As the sun set behind Bancroft Hall, you could feel the excitement and the anticipation building. Hundreds of boats, all sizes and types, were jockeying for a spot amidst an expressway of vessels that lined the harbor and the Severn. Barges on the Severn were in place, and fire department boats with red lights flashing formed a protective ring.

Following the sunset, a hazy purple light began to give way to darkness. The field lights shut off and the crowd erupted into cheers. Boats were blasting their air horns as a fever pitch of excitement built. Then, boom, boom, snap, crackle, boom, boom, the fireworks began. Brilliant, breathtaking explosions of color, thunderous booms and bangs shuddered right through me. Those are my favorites, the louder the better.

Screeching like a five-year-old, I dared my eyes and ears to take it all in. Glenn, quietly taking my hand, said, "Calm down, Annie, you'll pop something!" But he was grinning too.

The first volley must have lasted five glorious, exhilarating minutes, more like a finale than a beginning. Horns were blaring in appreciation, and I added my piercing wolf whistle.

Some of the fireworks were new to me. One I had never seen before shot up into the air with a trail of gold arching high up into the sky, and then when it could go no farther, there was a piercing bang as a huge starburst of gold, like shooting stars, spread out and cascaded downward toward the water. I think it was my favorite.

Perched on the cabin roof, hose in hand in case of sparks, camera at the ready, together we watched the amazing bursts of daylight that for a few seconds illuminated hundreds of white hulled boats. A thirty-foot flag waving from a nearby mast gave me goose bumps. It was impossible to capture the grandeur on 35 mm, but the illusion will be there and so will the memories.

While most of Annie and Glenn's sailing odysseys allowed them to experience the joy of getting away from problems at home where reality could be painful and depressing, they couldn't entirely escape tragedy and sadness even on their beloved Chesapeake.

We went into Annapolis on Saturday and lunched at Pussers on the bulkhead. We had whizzed by it for years and finally decided to go there. It was expensive and the food was just okay, so once was enough. We couldn't face going into our favorite pub, Biordens. We would keep expecting Carolyn to come out of the kitchen, blond hair bouncing, sweet smile, eyes sparkling in welcome. "Hi, sailors, welcome back, I know, potato skins, tuna melt—how are you?"

I haven't been able to write about her yet; I guess now is the time. I am in shock and disbelief that Carolyn O'Neil, our friend for fifteen years, is gone.

We met when we were at Biordens for the first time, and she had just been newly hired that week. We had brought Freyja to Horn Point and were discovering Annapolis. She suggested that we "must have potato skins" and we were hooked.

Over the years our friendship deepened and not just as waitress/patron. We kept in touch during the winter, Christmas mostly. She was always very caring and concerned over me when she felt I ordered the wrong thing.

She was so excited this Christmas, getting married to Nick, her long-term boyfriend. Her long-sought-after degree in elementary education was finally completed, and she had a teaching job secured for fall. "I'm on my way now, Annie!"

Carolyn was married in January. The Lord called her home in March—blood clot in her brain. She fainted at Biordens and died peacefully the next day.

We came in Biordens with the gang of our friends on a Saturday in May and asked for Carolyn.

Cindy gulped and said, "She's not on tonight, Annie." We found out later that the waitresses had gathered in the kitchen and decided not to tell us then. It was a busy Saturday night—a party, etc.—and we were with friends.

We bounded in Wednesday night and asked, "Hey, where's our girl?" Cindy looked at us, "Oh, Annie, Glenn, I'm so sorry, Carolyn died." Fighting back tears, I just stared, disbelieving. "No...No..." I then raced upstairs, followed by Glenn. Oh God, why? She was just getting started, married only six weeks. "Why, damn you, why her?" She was a giver, a caretaker, a nurturer to all who knew her. Andy came up sharing my sobs, telling me about the funeral. "Literally hundreds of people were there; she touched a lot of lives. There was no money for expenses, so the crew organized a fair and raised seven thousand dollars." I held onto Glenn, his eyes rimmed with tears. I threw down a rum and coke to stop shaking. The waitresses, bless their hearts, came over one by one telling me more. "She didn't suffer; we still miss her."

We picked our way through dinner, staring out the window, not looking into the pub. The image of Carolyn working her way through the tables, joking, smiling, was still too strong. We donated to her fund, got Nick's address, and stumbled out.

I prayed and talked to her because I know she is an angel now. It has taken a week to assimilate it all. My talk with a friend helped, telling me some of us aren't born to live long lives. They are here *as teachers, touching many in good and truthful living; their seemingly untimely death is yet another lesson.*

Jay, Glenn's brother, with his stirring example of abiding faith, never once questioned or showed anger at his fateful diagnosis of brain cancer. He accepted God's will and was filled with grace and courage like I had never seen. He died peacefully, without any pain, even though doctors said he would have horrible pain toward the end.

Carolyn, dear friend, you were and are a teacher. Your kindness, caring, and humor will not be forgotten. You are an example of tenacity, beating the odds and working your way through school to attain your dream. I'm so glad you did know the bliss of marriage and the fulfillment of receiving your degree. In death you teach me still. Life is fragile. Each day, whatever the circumstances, should be seized and cherished. Yesterday is but a memory. Tomorrow a dream to be sought, but today is ours, a reality that we make. No matter what tragedy or grief befalls us, we live and the storm shall pass. Life goes on around us. We must bounce back off the ropes of fate and go to the center of the ring to fight one more round.

I'm the one who should be dead, not you. My doctor said, "Anne, your gut is closing down. Surgery is the only option and very risky. You have about three weeks before your gut will be completely closed. I don't know how you are even eating now.

I could not get the catheter in your stoma more than one inch after an hour of trying. Never have I seen anything like it. I'm sorry, Anne."

That speech is ringing in my ears. Now one year later, I am not only eating, but gaining weight for the first time in twenty years! I can eat anything, the pain is a bit tough at times, but morphine helps and I'm on my way.

Why has the Lord healed me? What does he want me to do with this renewed life? The search for answers continues. I know I'm not strong enough to teach again. Perhaps I'm looking too hard for something too big. Maybe it is as simple as being a caretaker or being there for those I love, my family. I am blessed with such wonderful nieces and nephews whose devotion and love have pulled me through more than one nightmare.

We may never have money or a lot of material things but God has blessed us so. Loving each other deeply, I can still look at Glenn and well up with tears for the sheer joy of loving him. Of course there are times too when I could beat him with a frying pan.

Sailing had become so much more than a hobby, or an escape, or a sport, or a passion, that at one point, due to a challenging situation, they experimented with living aboard their boat year-round.

Incredibly, here we are in Annapolis living aboard Freyja in the middle of winter. Long underwear and sweats have replaced shorts and tank tops! Electric heaters are buzzing instead of fans.

Guess I should backtrack a bit and explain why we are here. This game show called "life" has taken a surprising but not unpleasant turn. Somehow I feel like we are being propelled along by an unseen force. Surely when I began to really trust in the Lord, our lives took a real swing toward our dream of living aboard.

Work in our area had dried up, but Glenn found out that there was ample work on boats in Annapolis and he could live aboard Freyja. It seemed to be at least a temporary answer to our money problems, although it meant that we would have to separate. I stayed in the cabin taking care of the animals and our home while Glenn lived on the boat and worked in Annapolis and came home as often as he could. Months went by like this but in the end I just couldn't stand to remain separated, so I found someone who would stay in the cabin and take care of the animals that I couldn't bring with me and I went to Annapolis to live with Glenn on the boat.

And now, again, the Lord has provided an answer. I truly feel empowered by the simple act of trusting in Him. Though our "stability," our home, is on permanent spin cycle, I am firmly rooted in my love for Glenn and my faith.

Living on Freyja gives me a contented, cozy feeling and time to reflect and reorganize. A heather pink sky with tufts of night purple clouds framed the scarlet sun this morning as I peeked over the blue coverlet. What a way to start the day. The morning chill disappeared as I breathed in the beautiful dawn. Thank you, Lord. I am still relishing just being here while shaking off the effects of being bedridden for nine months last year. I remember lying in bed so many times ready to scream for the want of just moving and breathing fresh air, to feel the wind on my face, desperate to just be outside.

Glenn is absolutely thrilled with his job. He is walking tall again with enthusiasm for each day. After a long workday, he comes aboard with a twinkle in his eye. He gets out his work log, and while drinking coffee, he proudly records each task while explaining it in detail and adding up each hard-earned dollar.

The future is definitely uncertain but so were all our yesterdays, and the challenge of having unknown horizons is stimulating and exciting. What sheer joy there is from just plain living and allowing time to become a friend instead of an adversary.

There is a right time and place for everything it seems, and after living on *Freyja* for a year, they realized that although they had enjoyed that life, they missed their cabin and being able to take in animals in need and rehabilitate them back to their natural life in the wild. It was also better for Annie to be closer to her doctors. Work for Glenn had become available in Cape May, so they resumed their life with the cabin being their home and getting away as much as possible to enjoy their sojourns on *Freyja*.

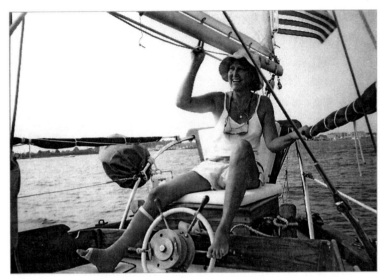

Now that's ingenuity!

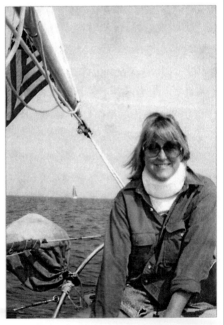

Not much kept Annie from sailing

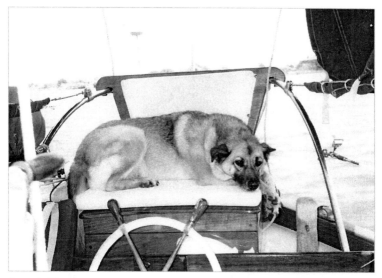

Captain Tippy

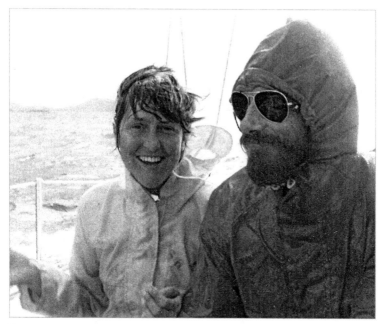

Thank goodness for wet gear!

CHAPTER TEN

Entre Nous

Up at 6:00 a.m. on a June day to watch the day begin. I can hear the gentle putt-putt of a crab boat as it passes in the darkness. A heron takes flight, cranky at being disturbed. The sky is thick with pewter clouds, but a hint of the sunrise is becoming evident in a light peach hue off to the starboard.

Glenn stirs beside me; a mosquito is bothering him and he opens his eyes briefly. I smile and say, "A new day is starting."

"Um-hmm-mm" is his groggy reply as he rolls over, burrowing deeper into the warm berth. I debate joining him, but decide to get coffee on. Maybe we'll have an early start today.

There is quite a chill in the air. I am sweat-suited from head to toe with socks and hood up.

My clanking and banging awakens Glenn. He takes over coffee duty, and I settle in for some quiet Bible time. I have decided to read the Bible on through— Genesis to Revelations. Maybe it will help give some direction to my understanding. I learned there are sixty-six books by forty-four men over a period of two centuries.

About an hour after we left shore, I went below for a head stop, and what should I find but the floorboards almost ready to float. I jumped into the cockpit and pumped my arm off. There was something definitely amiss. The water was pouring into the stern in the back of the engine. Glenn lowered the main to stop heeling, and the flow ceased. So the seam that has popped is above the waterline anyway. There is a chance that Glenn can fix it when we anchor. It would really be trouble if we were unable to sail because of water rushing in when she heels even 10 degrees. Damn and double damn. I know, I know . . . at least we are on the Chesapeake and on Freyja, but what a major, major disappointment if we can't even raise her sails, especially with Pops coming down. My fingers are crossed that the seam can be fixed. Ol' Pollyanna me, with the glass half full, will not let this hinder our time together.

We are cautiously entering Tilghman Creek now with the knowledge that our friend, Barry, spent four hours aground here. It is noon; the air is still and becoming progressively warmer. Layers of clothing are being peeled off. I'm down to shorts and a T-shirt. We have decided to pull into a nice little cove to port. It is the same spot we came to when we had Wendy and Linda aboard with us.

We all had quite a memorable night on that trip when a violent squall hit. We lost anchor and were headed toward the rocks. We had settled down for the night when a horrendous thunderstorm hit. I kept popping out of the companionway for the vicarious thrill of being out in the squall. The boat was rocking and lightning was crashing, lighting up the whole cove with an eerie gray intensity. We had awakened to an ominous pull and rapid movement of the boat. Hippie got up and went to turn off the depth meter.

Then all hell broke loose. The storm was blasting full tilt with a driving horizontal rain. Glenn bounded out of the companionway, started the engine, and yelled for a flashlight. He raced over the cabin top to grab the anchor that had drifted out. We were ten feet from the rocky shore going broadside with lightning and thunder crashing all around us and then the engine stalled. I dashed over to start the motor again. To my horror, the key broke off in the ignition.

Wendy was up by this time and came running to our assistance wearing nothing but a T-shirt and undies and was quickly sent to get the second key. Then Linda appeared topside in a short little nightie, still groggy from partying and blithely stepped in the middle of mayhem saying, "What's going on, why is Glenn pounding on the front deck?"

Trying not to be engulfed by the panic that was sweeping over me and scared for Glenn with the lightning, I was rain drenched and so fucking cold that I was shaking from head to foot. Wendy returned with the extra key and tweezers, and we scrunched down in the pouring rain, trying to pull out broken pieces of the key.

Meanwhile, Glenn was frantically trying to set the tiny anchor, which is like holding a cruise ship with a Danforth. Tension and terror were mounting with each bolt of lightning. Thunder, sounding like crashing cymbals, was all around us.

Then through the din we heard the most beautiful sound, the steady hum of an outboard motor coming our way. Our savior was a gentleman from a Canadian boat anchored nearby. He braved the downpour after hearing our panic-stricken voices. Linda, clad in soaked-through baby doll pj's gamely grabbed the anchor and stepped into the dinghy next to our rather embarrassed rescuer. She helped set the bow anchor while Glenn set the other one, all of which took about a half hour. We were all soaked and slightly freaked out.

We profusely thanked our rescuer and gave him a bottle of rum. The lightning provided an eerie silhouette as he motored away from us. All ended well.

I'm sure he had a tale to tell about the time he helped rescue a man with a three-girl crew dressed only in scant, wet nighties in the middle of a full-out squall.

Somehow I have to find a phone to call Pops and make sure all is set for Tuesday. I can't wait to have him aboard. He has had an incredibly tough haul this year. Being on the Chesapeake will refresh him, he does love it so. I need to remind him to bring his songbook. Glenn gets absolutely mortified when we start singing at the top of our lungs, but he shares in the joy of having Pops aboard.

After breakfast tomorrow we will go to my long-awaited bookstore, Lazy Moon. It is a treasure trove of old books and always transports me. I could browse there for hours! There is nothing like that wonderful, musty smell of old books, treasures of our heritage, between well-worn covers. Glenn, dear Glenn, waits on the porch with a cat in his lap looking out over the river. The last time we were there I found Uncle Wiggly and His Automobile *in its original dust jacket, the companion volume to Longfellow's* Evangeline, *stories for young women circa 1900, a little tell tale book,* Sailboat That Ran Away, *circa 1950, and a book about gnomes that was such a thrill. I have always wanted one, ever since my childhood, which has come more to my mind since Pops is due for a visit.*

Annie's father, "Pops" as she called him, was entering the later stages of his life and watching many things around him deteriorate, including the health of his mother,

Annie's beloved Gramma; the health of his wife, Bobbie; and the condition of his house and property, Fivormor. Both illnesses were a terrific strain for him, and Annie was frustrated because she didn't really have any way to help. Bobbie was depressed and Pops grew more and more lonely because he and Bobbie didn't go out any more, and so their life settled into a dull routine with little spontaneous joy. Pops was also troubled deeply by an ever-worsening financial picture. Although this was the time in his life when he should have been able to relax and enjoy the fruits of forty-five years of hard work, he had made some bad investment decisions and now it was all slipping away.

Annie had mixed feelings about Pops, all of which ran very deeply. When she saw him in the midst of a depressing lifestyle while she was enjoying such beauty while sailing, she came up with the plan to invite him down for a getaway weekend, hoping that sun and good wind could provide a break for him.

Awoke to a cold, mist-enshrouded dawn. We were completely surrounded by a heavy morning fog. Only the treetops were visible, poking their heads through to say good morning. A pink glow over the meadow was announcing the sunrise, and as the rays filtered through the trees the cotton candy fog took on a rosy glow and began to rise, rushing ahead of the dawn's warmth.

I am so excited. We are on our way to pick up Pops! I changed the V-berth, and with lint flying, I played clothesline, flapping sheets in the breeze to freshen them.

It has turned into a clear and beautiful day. We dropped hook in St. Mike's and Pops arrived at 9:30 on the dot. What joy to finally get him aboard. Following that we motor sailed up to cousin Patsy's. She waved us on in along with Wye, a black Lab who delighted in literally diving for oysters, and Rosey, a striking young Setter who gamely tried to join in the fun but was a bit confused. They were then joined by their neighbor, a Chesapeake retriever named Alice. They all had quite an afternoon romping in the water. I have never seen dogs dive underwater then sit up and beg, tracking bottom with their hind legs. What a comical sight to behold.

We spent a lovely afternoon jes settin' under the trees, Pops and his dear cousin reminiscing about times past. Patsy really is a happy soul with a ready smile and a down-home personality. Her home sits right across from Drum Point. What a spectacular view, clear all the way to St. Mike's!

It was a treat to visit with her and hear stories of Pops, her "cousin Phil," who seemingly was often in the midst of all kinds of mischief. I especially loved seeing her home, cluttered with family antiques. Pops and Patsy, both talking at once and barely stopping for a breath, had a grand time identifying family in the wonderful Heaver-Tyler-Edgerton album.

Turning those worn black pages filled with small brown-and-white pictures takes you back to a peaceful era. Boys in knickers and girls in white frocks posed with self-conscious grins by a small hedge. A family picture was taken on Uncle John's porch.

"Now that's my grandmother, Alice, and there's my grandfather, Jack, teasing Frances," Cousin Patsy remembered. "Oh, how he loved to kid your Gramma. She was kind of shy and he would say, 'Hi, honey bun' just to see her blush. Oh, she loved him so; and that's Daisy, she was married to Sam Edgerton over there. They had nine children; all died save one, little Dorothy right there. And that, Phil, who's that? Oh, that's your great-grandmother, such a sense of humor, always smiling. And Nellie, dear Nellie and Parker."

Stories were tenderly remembered, passed down from generation to generation. Words came tumbling out so fast, and I remembered Gramma's voice pointing to these same pictures and remembering "back then" and laughing at such happy times.

It was such a confusing feeling, knowing Gramma wasn't doing well at home, yet knowing that this is the cycle of life turning forward all the time. How could I be morose when in the presence of Cousin Patty? She is such a character, full of pep and relishing in the sheer joy of the moment.

With stomachs growling, we reluctantly said good-bye around 4:30. We motored on up to Dividing Creek to drop our hook and had a lazy night. We ate steak, noodles, and beans under the stars and giggled 'cause we couldn't quite see what we were eating.

The wind started to put quite a chill on our stargazing efforts, so we went below to turn in. I tucked Pops in. It was a rather comical proceeding because he had forgotten to bring warm pants so he put flannels on over his preppy red ones and then added a gargantuan winter goose down parka. He looked like a veritable puffball.

All snug now, we slept soundly, looking forward to spending another day together.

Annie's idea of a respite for Pops worked, but he then had to return to watch over Gramma after this brief reprieve. Annie's heart was with Gramma and Pops, and she would call for updates, which grew worse all the time. Her phone calls with Pops—he in his neglected, run-down house, and she at a random pay phone from some marina—would end up with both of them in tears. Then, one of them would suggest they sing a hymn together, and they would do so in broad voices regardless of where she was at the time.

I know I will never truly be without her. Gramma's presence is woven into the fabric of my life. Pictures of our joyous times together are forever etched in my memory. The depth and strength of her love, a mother's love, comforts me. The witness to the seeds of faith she planted and nurtured within me are flowering even now when I feel despair, witnessed as I reach for the scripture, searching for comfort in God's word. Tears blur the words as I see her notes and touch her fingerprints on the faith-worn pages of her Bible. Keepsakes from Gramma are pressed between its pages, notes and drawings sent to cheer me over the years. The "Armor of God" is my favorite, sent to me while I was in the hospital. It was taken from Ephesians 6:14–17 and depicts a knight in full gear, hood of salvation, girdle of the truth, mantle of righteousness, armed with the sword of the spirit and word of God, protected by a shield of faith, fending off fiery arrows. The sentiment so dear reads, "With trembly loving hands for my precious Annie, I love you so much, you have brought joy to my life."

She loved me as a mother, without judgment or restraint. I felt strong and secure, pulling her love around me like a sweater, warm and reassuring. Images of Gramma flood my mind, making me sad, yearning for what has been, yet happy also, and comforting, like looking through photos in an album.

Gramma was ninety-seven and, as sadly expected, the phone call came that she had slipped into a coma.

Glenn understood how much Gramma meant to me and what an important influence she had on my life. He also understood that she gave me the only unconditional love that I had ever known until I met him.

Pops had a hard time at first accepting Glenn as the man that his daughter had fallen in love with, but this all changed as he got to know Glenn and his devotion to Annie.

> *Glenn, my precious, understanding husband, patiently puts up with Pops and me. He alone truly understands our relationship and is big enough to never resent it. God, he is a treasure.*

Annie's relationship with Pops was indeed highly complex. He could be so absorbed with his own life that he could forget her birthday, and then she would have to call to remind him. He would react with surprise and then get all flustered, muttering: "Oh damn!" But even in times when Pops was being self-centered and arrogant, she still knew that he loved her, which was evident from letters he wrote her, such as this one:

> *Dearest Anne,*
>
> *Just a note to tell you how happy I am for you.*
>
> *You and Glenn are going to find in planning your wedding that you will both be caught in some tugs and pulls 'tween our "interesting" family group. Be prepared to grin and bear it cuz in the end it'll all be carried out with lots of fun, moments to cherish and a lifetime of joy ahead.*
>
> *Love,*
> *Pops*

Annie's father recognized that there were problem dynamics within their family and that his wife had sided decisively with her children. Going against her wishes would have created dissension in their marriage, so even though he was very close with Annie, he had to keep many interactions with his daughter secret from Bobbie.

> *Dearest Anne,*
> *Here is my engagement present.*
> *I know you will want a few odds and ends for the big event.*
> *There are times when parents share certain secrets with their children.*
> *I do not condone too much subterfuge cuz it can be reasoned that it dwells on a fine line with dishonesty which I deplore, however me darling daughter, this little gifty is very strictly entre nous- very, very " " " " "!*
> *Love,*
> *Ol' Pop*

Annie knew all of his flaws, yet she also credited him for teaching her never to give up:

> *Surely you don't walk the path of IBD alone. Loyal and caring friends and family have been a constant source of encouragement and comfort.*
> *Early on, my father taught me to fight the odds. He never allowed me to give up on myself or be defeated by the flare-ups and surgeries that inevitably followed.*

I never would have had the courage to finish school or pursue a career without his constant support. He taught me that one person could truly make a difference in the lives of many. Refusing to accept the rather dismal prognosis, he fought despair with hope.

Through research, single-mindedly, he reorganized a faltering local NFIC chapter in Philadelphia, recruiting doctors and citizens to spread the word about IBD. He was successful in raising hundreds of thousands of dollars for research.

Words can't express how very much I cherish and love my dear, complicated, stubborn, sermonizing, intelligent, hymn-singing, gentle, loyal Pops. When he visits us aboard Freyja, it is like the past has been erased in some way, or the playing field has been leveled, and we are able to relate like peers or simply as two souls communing on the open water.

Once he gets his sea legs under him, he wakes me with a not-so-gentle yank on my hair. He has always been up since before dawn with coffee in one hand and the Bible in the other.

With Bobbie's health declining as surely as Gramma's, Pops had no choice but to put his wife in Bryn Mawr Hospital, thinking it was a nervous breakdown. Her blood pressure was dangerously high and she had severe body tremors plus a thirty-pound weight loss. The doctors kept her for a week, infusing her with phenobarbitol and visterol for a week before her blood pressure came down. Then came the final blow: she was told that she had to give up cigarettes; this after forty-five years of smoking. She became quite angry and hostile, especially to Pops, refusing to see anyone or accept phone calls.

Pops adopted a tone of bravado for Annie over the phone, but she knew how very worried he was. After all, he depended on Bobbie for so much; she really had been his best friend and companion. Annie convinced him to come spend some time once again on the boat, knowing it would relax and soothe him under the pressure of troubled finances, with both a wife and a mother who were ill.

> *Pops is rustling about so it's time to get up with him and watch the dawn. Pops read to me from* Upper Room, *a religious book of verses. We talked about the reality of Bible stories. He has a book of archaeology that is rousing questions of creation, i.e., how to reconcile science and religion. Gramma has such a pure and innocent faith. The Bible is the word and that is that. No doubts, no questions.*
>
> *We spent some time bird watching. Dad kept calling the egrets, ibis. We watched a heron fishing. He definitely has laid claim to this cove, barking and chasing away any other bird that dared to venture into his domain.*
>
> *Hopefully Pops is getting some respite from his troubles at home. As an extra treat, we ran into Uncle Tommy and brought him out to see Freyja. We spent a pleasant time reminiscing in the cockpit.*

Pops entertained us with yarns about Uncle Tommy and their boat, Onion. As teenagers, the cousins would take off in this open rowboat that was sloop rigged and provisioned with canned beans, tomatoes, and water. Good heavens, no Ziplocs, hot coffee, or steaks? And they call that cruising? Their nights were spent ashore. One night they took their blankets—no sleeping bags in those days—and bedded down in a pasture. Pops awoke with the eerie feeling of being watched. Ever so slowly he opened his eyes to find a big nose sniffing him curiously. The nose was attached to a rather bemused horse that was trying to decide what this prone figure was. Startled, Pops jumped, frightening the horse who took off like a shot with his thundering hooves echoing in Dad's ears.

He and Uncle Tommy spent many happy hours together on the Chesapeake. These surroundings hold a flood of memories for Pops, mostly of more carefree times. (Uncle Tommy told us the same horse story over lunch another time, but in his version, he was the one under the horse!)

When we awaken to a wet, foggy, solid, gray rainy day, we play gin rummy. Pops cracks me up with the ol' Heaver squint every time I knock. Boy, he does not like to lose, but he always beats me in the end.

Gad, I'm so disappointed for Pops. It is always so sad for me when I leave him on the dock waving good-bye, not knowing if this will be the last time he visits us aboard Freyja.

Then the bomb dropped. Pops told Annie there were shadows on Bobbie's most recent CAT scan. The dreaded word cancer finally was voiced. Pops was under such strain that he was refusing to really talk about what was happening. He finally only shared the pain because Annie kept bugging him.

She is home now and Pops is saying that it, meaning cancer, was a mistake. I don't believe him though. Bobbie is still losing weight. She finally did talk to me briefly, sounded so weak and still angry about no cigarettes. I have concluded that her attitude stinks and is pulling her down even further. I really want to write her a letter, to encourage and maybe comfort her, but I just don't know if it would help or make matters worse. I'm praying frantically for them both. It pulls my insides out to hear Pops.

I know it sounds hopelessly Pollyanna, but tough times can strengthen us. There is one unalterable freedom you always have no matter the physical circumstances. Your mind, your soul is free, free to choose how this chapter in your life will read.

There were many mornings in the hospital when I used to make a conscious choice. I could choose depression, give in to it and let the whole hospital experience wrap around me, which certainly would have been easier, or I could take the other road and fight against the overwhelming desire to cave in. Choosing this road I would plaster on a smile, drum up some humor, which is the best weapon and ally, and learn to be content in whatever situation I was in. Then sooner than you think you start to believe your Pollyanna attitude and find that others will respond in kind. If you are down, they will slide down too. It is a simple enough formula but very hard to practice at times.

To even speak these words to Pops makes me sound suspect, holier-than-thou, I know, yet he listens to me and respects my position even if it isn't one he can adopt fully right now. We all need to help keep each other strong and to remind each other that we have to choose to make the best of whatever state we are in.

What's done is done. What's been said has been said. We can't undo the mistakes of yesterday, but we can make sure that our behavior today doesn't contribute to unnecessary problems for tomorrow.

In spite of everything, I feel blessed that Pops and I have found a way to communicate our love for each other in a way that strengthens us both, at times delights us both, and in the end, redeems us both.

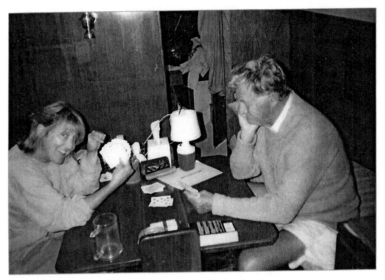

Pops did not like to lose at cards

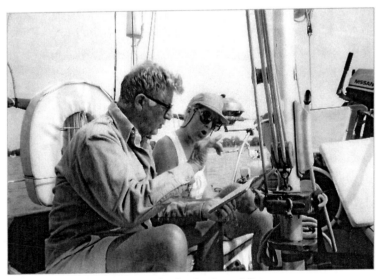

Singing hymns together was a joy for Annie and Pops

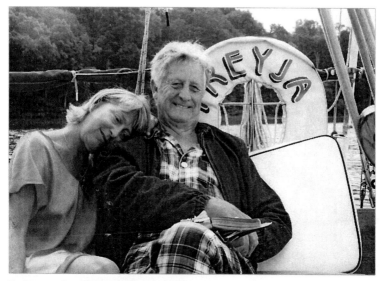

Early morning Bible time with Pops on *Freyja*

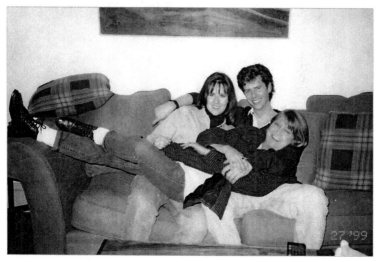

Annie being Annie with David and Lynnie

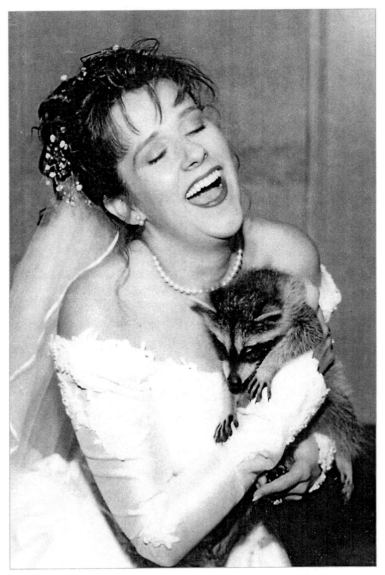

Baby Noah was a special guest at Lynnie's wedding

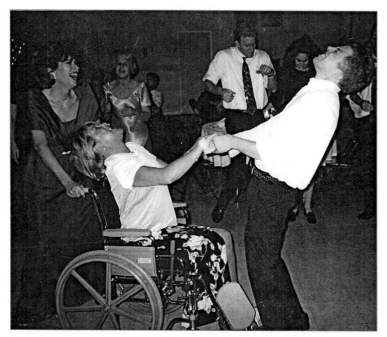

With one leg in a cast, Annie was wheelchair "dancing" at Lynnie's reception

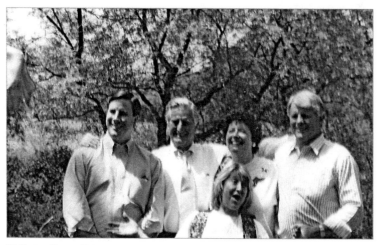

Phil, Jr., Pops, Tyler, and Lowrey standing behind Annie

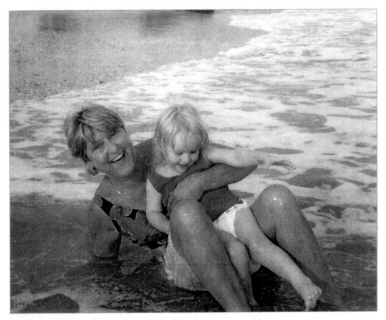

Annie playing in the waves with baby Heather, David's daughter

CHAPTER ELEVEN
A Great Comeback

※ ⁓ ※

ROLF BENIRSCHKE, former placekicker for the San Diego Chargers, first came up with the idea of the Great Comebacks Award. Rolf himself was diagnosed with life-threatening colitis at the age of twenty-four, during his second season in the National Football League. He had ostomy surgery in 1979, and went through what many men, women, and children go through in his situation: pain and embarrassment, the momentary desire to back away from life, and the misperception that their life, as they know it, is over.

"I woke up with an ileostomy [an ostomy related to the small intestine]," Rolf says, "and I wondered what the future held for me. I was just starting out in professional athletics, and it seemed my future was shut off.

"While I was in the hospital, I was visited by someone who had had an ostomy. He said I could do everything I could do prior to my surgery. I said, 'Yes, but I'm a professional athlete.'"

Despite Rolf's protests at the time, his belief in the words of his visitor grew as Rolf resumed playing tennis, found his way into wind surfing and skiing, and eventually returned to the football field. He notes that he had to do all of these things with a little more preparation, but he could do them. The important decision was the one to try. When Rolf earned his spot back on the team, he went on to have his best years in football after he returned. Rolf was named NFL Man of the Year in 1983.

"My comeback created a lot of media attention and prompted thousands of letters," Rolf has said. "Most of the letters began: 'You're the first person I heard of with the same illness I have. . . .'"

Realizing that there was a need for IBD sufferers to talk openly about their surgeries and their ostomies, Rolf went to ConvaTec (an international corporation that manufactures products for use in the areas of ostomy and wound care) with an idea. "Let's get out there and share the stories with your patients, that life is fine after surgery. Instead of being doomed because of an ostomy, you can now do things you couldn't do before, because now you're healthier."

That's how the Great Comebacks Award was created in 1984 by the National Foundation for Ileitis and Colitis (NFIC) for sufferers of ileitis and colitis. It celebrates those who have overcome seemingly impossible personal calamities and have gone on to lead productive lives. The obstacles may be formidable, but the rewards can be even greater because of them. The question is: Do we allow ourselves to be defeated by whatever fate has dealt us? Or do we take it as a challenge, a turning point, and come back stronger than ever?

All of her life, Annie had been inspiring her community with her determination to get back on her feet and live life to the fullest after each physical setback she endured. It amazed all who knew her how she was able to continue with such optimism when she spent so much of her time in hospitals with severe pain. When Annie was well, she went full speed ahead in life as if she had to recapture the time that had been taken away from her. All of her senses were put into overdrive to make the most out of every healthy minute. She used humor to soften even the worst of situations; sometimes her biggest calamities made the best stories. Her speech was animated, and her laugh was raucous, infectious, and frequent. Her listeners were captivated by her unique experiences and her zest for life.

Annie had an insatiable desire to help others, and she did so with honesty, compassion, and humor. Just as Rolf Benirshcke's visitor had shown him a door into the future where Rolf only saw a wall, Annie counseled IBD patients who, after undergoing ostomy surgery, could only see a bleak future for their lives. Oftentimes her visit to a scared, depressed young person would give the patient hope and the desire to get back into the life they had once cherished.

Waking up with an ostomy is a tremendous shock. It takes time and experience to adjust to this change.

The change in your self-image can be shattering, but you have to realize that it enables you to live. It does not change who or what you are. An ostomy doesn't mean your life is over. Ostomy surgery is a second chance at living, at a better quality of life. Your life will no longer be measured in terms of where the nearest bathroom is. You shouldn't be embarrassed about having such problems, and when other people are curious and concerned, the best thing is to explain it to them, again with humor. You can fight more easily with humor. It takes the sting out of embarrassing symptoms.

Annie would remind those who feared a loss of their sexuality that she was single when her first ostomy surgery was performed.

Sex appeal comes from within, from how we present ourselves. Your life will go on, and be even better. Once you get over the hurdle of having the pouch, you can do anything you did before. At first, after the ostomy surgery, you grieve. You have lost a part of your body, like losing an arm or a leg. You have to let yourself go through it. Yet after a while, you realize that you're the only one who can get yourself up and out.

Annie was quick to remind those whom she visited that people who have Crohn's disease shouldn't think that her medical history would be theirs. Her case was a very severe one and not representative of all people with Crohn's.

In the late summer of 1988, for example, she was working as an enrichment tutor with a marvelous boy who literally changed her life. He was a very gifted, special boy in the first grade, impish, witty and mischievous with blond good looks. Annie really came to adore him and had become wonderfully attached to his whole family.

She very badly wanted to teach again, to have purpose, meaning, and she worked hard preparing her materials, at least three to four hours per day. Her stamina took a nosedive and she finally had to admit that it was time to stop around Thanksgiving. The pain continued, and by Christmas, her weight loss had made her look like a ninety-pound refugee. Malnutrition and chronic pain are an all-too-familiar scenario for some IBD sufferers because of their inability to absorb enough nutrition to maintain weight. Annie ended up at the Hospital of the University of Pennsylvania two days before Christmas, her favorite holiday of all.

There it became obvious that Annie would need to receive hyperalimentation, a process that would allow her bowels to rest by having no food by mouth while receiving complete nutrition intravenously through a permanent catheter. Now, not all people with Crohn's need hyperalimentation if they have an ileostomy, nor do most people with Crohn's need an ileostomy. But Annie seemed selected for the special purpose of enduring the worst of what her disease had to offer.

A port-o-cath was surgically implanted between my boobs on our anniversary, lucky # 13 no less.

Glenn went through a tough adjustment period but has been so very loving and compassionate throughout. The whole business hit me very hard. There were days of denial and tears of disbelief. BUT, the weight gain has really been beneficial, hindsight as usual, making things easier. Dear and precious caring friends buoyed us up. My little student came with his whole family, bringing a wreath and Christmas decorations, and other friends arrived on New Year's Day replete with huge banners that said 'Soar with Eagles.' Our anniversary banners on January 17 had a picture of us "dancing," with me attached to pumps. We truly are blessed with loving and loyal friends.

It was during this hospital stay that the Philadelphia chapter of the National Foundation for Ileitis and Colitis approached Annie believing that she would be a good candidate for the Great Comebacks Award. They knew that the Great Comebacks Award was looking for people who had crossed that mental and emotional bridge in their lives into acceptance and went on to achieve their goals. They believed Annie was a great candidate for the program as she was willing to share her stories with others who were battling the same disease, and so a representative came to visit Annie in the hospital a few weeks after surgery with an application in hand. Because Annie was still too weak to write, she dictated her story into a microphone that Glenn held for her for a few minutes at a time over a period of several days.

*I taped my story for the "Great Comebacks" appli-
cation while tubed and bottled. I really didn't feel
like being a Pollyanna, but questions made me
reflect on all the positive influences and events
over the tumultuous pathways of this disease. I
was really too ill to write much, so Glenn, to the
rescue once again, tape recorded most of it. Dear
Jennifer Reynolds, a representative from the NFIC
Philadelphia chapter, transcribed it for me and
mailed in the application, a seemingly simple deed
that has changed my life.*

The application was sent in, and with the passing of
time Annie forgot about it as she continued to recover and
gain strength. The weight gain afforded by the considerable inconvenience of receiving hyperalimentation turned
out to be very beneficial, with Annie's stamina and pain
tolerance increasing daily.

One day Annie was recuperating at home when the
phone call came. It was Rolf Benirschke telling Annie that
she had been selected out of hundreds of applicants as the
winner of this year's Great Comebacks Award. He told her
that it was Tip O'Neil, the Speaker of the House, who was
the first one to read Annie's story and said, "This is it, this
is the one!" The rest of the committee then read Annie's
story, and all of them agreed that she was an exceptional
candidate and indeed the perfect one to share her inspirational and moving story.

Following the phone call, Rolf sent Annie a letter saying in part, "You really do have a tremendous story to tell,

and we are looking forward to working with you to help get the word out to others who are struggling with IBD or ostomy surgery that there is a light at the end of the tunnel!"

Enclosed was a promotional release form for "The Turning Point," a newsletter that was published twice a year in which they planned to feature Annie's story. Rolf also notified Annie that an advertising agency would be getting in touch with her regarding the details for her trip to New York, which would include photo shoots and a media tour. An entire three-day weekend in June had been planned out where Annie would be honored, receive her award, and give an acceptance speech. Suddenly Annie was a celebrity!

After Annie was released from the hospital, hyper-alimentation was delivered to her cabin from Caremark Homecare. As Annie described it, "Four times a week, for fourteen hours a day, I hook myself up to my own personal R2D2. I guess I've known all along that hyperalimentaion was in my future, because I have only four feet of ileum (small intestine) left, creating short bowel syndrome and an inability to absorb nutrition."

An article about Annie was published in the *Mid Atlantic Currents* at that time, written by Pete LaBerge. Excerpts from the article read as follows:

> *A squall was racing down the Delaware Bay as I entered Anne Stites's log cabin in Cape May Court House, New Jersey. "Wait until you see this, Pete! You'll love it," said Anne. She put the coffee on and within minutes, the skies opened up with lightning*

cracking all around. The lovely cabin, built by her husband, Glenn, from huge telephone poles, was fast becoming an island amid the pines.

The animals had mixed feelings about the storm. Mac the parrot said hello to anyone who would listen. Moose, part husky, hid under a table while Scupper, a big, droopy bassett hound nuzzled my feet. Tilly, the ferret, investigated a plastic bag, while Pepper, the forty-three-pound raccoon was, thankfully, behind closed doors upstairs. Did I mention that Anne and Glenn love animals?

The squall passed quickly and we continued to talk about Anne's tutoring of "special" children. She had to overcome many obstacles to receive her degree; now she shares her gifts in teaching and counseling whenever she is able. At forty, Anne has lived with Crohn's disease since seventh grade. After twenty-three operations, including fifteen resections, Anne continues to have difficulty absorbing nutrients. Since starting hyperalimentation with Caremark two months ago, Anne has gained weight and continues to feel better physically.

She will need all her energy for a very important weekend next month! On June 18, a limo will whisk Anne and Glenn from their rustic cabin to the glittering canyons of New York City. On June 20, Anne will be presented with the Steuben crystal eagle by the National Foundation of Ileitis and Colitis as the recipient of the 1989 Great Comebacks Award.

> *Anne is a little worried about what she will say in New York but I'm not. She speaks effortlessly about her life, her hopes and her dreams in spite of her disease. I feel that I have known her for years.*
>
> *Anne is an optimist from whom we could all take lessons. She is confident that a cure for Crohn's and IBD will come someday. In the meantime, her inspiring advice echoes in my head as I leave for home, "Don't give up on your dreams and your goals. You may have to alter your course, but GO FOR IT!"*

Annie continued gaining weight and strength in the months following her surgery as she thought about preparing for the biggest weekend of her life. She ruminated over everything from what she would say to what she would wear, a touching display of self awareness for a woman whose life was so entirely devoted to others. But after all, she explained, there were going to be dinners and interviews for newspapers, radio, and TV . . . and then there was the luncheon where she would receive her award and speak in front of more than 600 people! Annie went through her entire wardrobe and came to the conclusion that not one piece of it would do for such an important weekend, and so the shopping spree began.

Glenn found it unbelievable that Annie could find such joy in going from store to store and trying on one outfit after another. It seemed to him that she would not be able to complete her mission until she had tried on every article of clothing that was available within a ten-mile radius of their cabin. Annie's endurance would give out after about two hours, and the search for the perfect clothes would have to be postponed until the next day. With his usual persona, Glenn was her companion, carrying the bags and quietly enduring the whole ordeal while Annie was bursting with excitement and vivaciously chatting with sales ladies. Even Glenn did not escape, as he was himself outfitted with pleated pants, one cream color, one khaki, a blue sports coat, socks, and shirts.

The carefully selected outfits were hung in the den and just looking at them filled Annie with a flood of emotions in anticipation for the weekend that would soon be arriving. She had had fragments of ideas for her speech running around in her head for weeks. She had pages and pages of ideas. She went back and forth trying out various metaphors, mixing her natural nervousness with her very real desire to get her words right.

There was an analogy about a squirrel in her notes, for example:

> ... the squirrel was clamoring up a pole to reach the feeder full of food only to find a Plexiglas square blocking his way. The squirrel tried for more than an hour going up and down the pole, then finally one last bang on the glass and at last he sat triumphantly inside the full feeder. He had reached his goal. How many times I had felt like that squirrel with my goal in sight, only then to have a flare-up or surgery and slide back down the pole. But unlike the squirrel, I had help getting back up that pole.

When the day came to leave for New York, her speech still lay unwritten. There were so many thoughts of gratitude and love that she found it hard to express everything in one place. Fortunately, her health was intact; after a warm spring, Annie was looking and feeling well. She was tan and had gained twenty pounds, coming back from a low weight of ninety pounds.

Thursday, June 18, finally arrived, and thus commenced Annie and Glenn's odyssey, what she joked should be referred to as "Ma and Pa Kettle go to the Big City." A shiny black stretch limo turned down Highs Beach Road, a half-mile-long, wooded road that dead-ends at the beach—it was a good bet that this was the first time a limousine had ever been down there! The cabin is not visible from the road, but sighting the "Stites Boat Work" sign, the driver turned into the dirt and grass driveway. The limo, looking incongruous in its setting, quickly reached a parking area in front of a split rail fence faced with turkey wire to keep the animals inside.

Passing through the gate, the driver was met by two dogs happy to see a visitor. He continued down a brick path and through an arbor leading to the cabin. The driver, Nick, a real "New Yoiker" who never before had been sent to such a unique home and property, was enthralled with the charming, rustic setting of the hand-built log cabin.

Annie, who was so excited, chatted with Nick all the way up to the Grand Hyatt, which turned out to be aptly named. It had a huge lobby and marble steps and three stories of flowers with people milling all around. Shops with brass lights shone on mirrored walls. The VIP manager escorted Annie and Glenn to their room, which was actually a suite. Glenn was in heaven—they had two bathrooms! Even the walk-in closets were huge; Glenn hid in one and kept calling Annie's name while she ran around in circles laughing and trying to find him.

They put their feet up for all of ten minutes and then dressed for dinner with Mickey and Wendy, a nice couple from advertising who had come down to the cabin for an interview a few weeks ago. After that they were off to the show, *Me and My Girl*, a musical comedy that Annie had requested. She had said, "How can we be in New York City and not see a musical?"

They pulled up to the theater in a chauffeur-driven limousine and Annie felt like Cinderella going to the ball. In a most moving way, she soaked up every second of this magical night. It was inevitable that the excruciating pain would return, and that this surreal fairytale would become a pleasant mental oasis to which she could return in the many dark days to come.

Glenn, as befits his character, was a little bit embarrassed by all of the attention. He thought it was ridiculous that they would be chauffeured to the theater when it was within walking distance!

Annie and Glenn had been given third-row seats and could actually see the actors sweat. The staging was beautiful and the choral numbers, dazzling. Forty-second Street was a mob scene afterward. They looked and looked for their limo to no avail, finally hopping into a battered old cab that reeked of incense. As they passed the Marriot, they spotted their name card in the window of a black long stretch limo. "Stop!" Annie yelled and together they scrambled out leaving one befuddled driver for another as they leapt into their luxurious limo. This ride had a TV, a telephone, climate control, a bar, and a moon roof. The car was so long that they had to use a telephone to talk to the driver!

They tumbled into bed around 12:30 a.m. with Annie unable to sleep because there were phrases from her unwritten speech dancing in her head. Panic was beginning in earnest now!

The next day they were roused by a wake-up call at 6:30 a.m., with coffee and the newspaper waiting by the door. They ordered a sumptuous breakfast from room service—Annie was off hyperalimentation by this time and back to eating normally—while a hairdresser, makeup artist, and media consultant tried to get Annie ready for her interviews that would begin at 10:00 a.m. Annie recalled, "They made me look like I was going on *American Bandstand*, thick, black eyeliner, with my hairdo a bit 'high.' I told them I was getting an eagle but I didn't want to look like one!" Annie's media consultant, Rori, came to her aid, admonishing the makeup artist, "Now, Leon, she's from the country and not used to all that!" Annie rushed to the bathroom, trying in vain to rub off some of the eye paint. But they were running late—it was three minutes to the radio interview!

During Annie's first radio interview, Rolf Benirschke walked into the media room.

My heart skipped twelve beats. He is strikingly hand-some—khakis, polo shirt, and a sweater draped over his shoulders. He chatted with Glenn, then came over, bent down, and gave me a kiss. There went my interview! "Whoops, Barb, can you tape that part over?!" When the interview was finished, Rolf said, "Now, how about a real hug." He is so very nice; I felt at ease in the first few minutes! He was there to get his interview schedule, which was a full day for him, CBS, ABC. He had just flown in from the West Coast.

Next a reporter from Newsday arrived, a tall, lanky, hippie-looking young man, who asked very thoughtful and sensitive questions: "What made you want to keep getting up?" "I can see one, two, or even three surgeries but how did you feel after twenty-three?!" He was incredulous and sympathetic.

Annie answered the questions as best as she could. She said that her strengths came through faith and love for her precious Glenn. She knew in the very depth of her being that she had to get better, to live her life with Glenn. The thought of giving up rarely entered her mind. There were many painful, lonely nights, nightmarish tests, and indescribable pain—yet her blessings always seem to overshadow the despair. She preferred to center on the many positive aspects of her life, such as her loving and loyal family, including her dear Pops who first taught her never to give in to this disease, to fight the odds, to have faith. Their sunrise phone calls continued to this day, Annie told the reporters. Her Pops's voice, "Hi ya, sweet potato—how was your night?" It was so comforting to have a sympathetic voice in the gray, early morning hours.

The interviews continued throughout the day. There were people standing by ready to freshen Annie's makeup and bring her food and beverages. Some interviews were taped over the phone and some were face-to-face. The last one was videotaped for NBC. Later, Annie would receive a letter from an old classmate from Ithaca College that read in part, "While puttering around my living room, I happened to look up while Carol Jenkins of *NBC News* conducted an interview with a very familiar face. To my delight I discovered it was my college dorm mate from Ithaca College. It has been almost twenty years, but I have often remembered you and wondered how you were. It was heartwarming to see that you had been honored and looked so radiant!"

By the time the interviews were over, there was no time for rest—the cocktail party in Annie's honor was to begin at four-thirty! So many people wanted to meet her, this courageous woman with the indomitable spirit who had, in spite of her severe disease, given so much to other people to make their lives better. She received hugs and congratulations from a room full of people, stars in their own right.

Returning to their suite, Annie realized how exhausting the day had been. She needed to sleep and dozed off until her eyes popped open the next morning at the break of dawn.

My speech, Oh my God, my speech!
I quickly got out of bed and went to the table that held a stack of papers that were strewn in disarray, obviously not in any decided order.

"Okay, this is it," I said to myself. "No more time, I need to complete this now."

I sat down with note cards and after some time sorting through all of my papers, began to write. I wrote while Glenn slept. I kept writing and organizing. Sometime later I sat back and said, "Well, that's it." I had written a dozen or more cue cards and put them in order, finally convinced that even if my efforts were not good enough, they were my best efforts after all.

We ordered breakfast from room service, more modestly than the day before, and I laid out my outfit and accessories. Glenn got up and tried to calm me, his anxious wife. "You can do this, Annie," he said. "You'll be great. If you get nervous, I'll be there, just talk to me."

Makeup and hair arrived for the glamour treatment, and just after Annie had finished dressing, the ad person knocked on the door to take them downstairs to meet with the press and photographers for an hour before the luncheon. They were led to a room that was filled with press from radio and TV stations, celebrities, and important people from the NFIC. After about half an hour they were shuffled off into another room where photographers were waiting to photograph Annie for the newspapers and magazines.

Then, after months of preparing and anxiously waiting, it seemed that the moment arrived quite suddenly. They were to be ushered into the Empire State Ballroom at the

Grand Hyatt Hotel. Annie hesitated at the door, stunned for a moment when she saw the room filled with more than 600 people, all there to meet her and hear her speak. This place in time felt surreal. After all of the imagining how it would actually feel, here she was. Seeing her hesitation Glenn squeezed her hand. "Come on, honey, they're waiting for you," he said. "This is why we're here."

Annie was escorted to the head table while Glenn was shown to the next ranking table of celebrities and found his place card next to Marvin Bush, the current president's youngest son. Actress and former Miss America, Mary Ann Mobley and her husband, television personality, Gary Collins, were on his other side.

People settled at the round tables of ten, and lunch was served while a few remarks were made by representatives of the award's sponsors, ConvaTec and NFIC. Neither Glenn nor Annie ate a mouthful of food. Glenn was too nervous and Annie didn't dare eat, fearing that her ostomy bag would fill up and the appliance would possibly break.

Once the luncheon dishes had been cleared, Rolf got up and went to the podium to announce the 1989 winner of the Great Comebacks Award. He spoke for several minutes briefly covering Annie's background and medical history and why she had been selected out of so many applicants to win this prestigious award. He wanted everyone to know the full amount of devastation that she and her body had been through in her forty years of life, in case she didn't address these facts. In his eyes, he said, it made her story that much more remarkable.

Rolf concluded with, "And now I would like to introduce to you this remarkably courageous winner of the 1989 Great Comebacks Award, Anne Stites." There was applause as Annie rose from her chair, making eye contact with Glenn at the next table. He smiled and gave her the thumbs-up signal, something he did just before every surgery.

Gathering her note cards, she took a deep breath and walked to the podium in front of hundreds of people who were applauding and waiting to hear what she had to say.

She took a few moments to look at her notes and realized with some degree of panic that with the glare of the lighting and her not-so-perfect eyesight, she couldn't read what she had written. She took another moment to calm herself down and assured herself that she knew what she wanted to say, what message she wanted to get across, and that she didn't need notes to do it. So, with her incredible ability to accept and adapt to changes in her life, she quickly decided to forgo the notes and just speak from her heart.

Annie began to talk. I have never heard anyone speak who had quite the ability to capture and move people like Annie could. The minutes went by and there wasn't a sound in the room except Annie's voice.

She didn't go into her agonizing life of (then) twenty-three surgeries and long, painful recoveries. She talked about how you can go on living in spite of them, making every day that you are not in pain count. She talked about how you could get back on your feet and handle your disease with honesty and humor. She talked about how you could find joy and fulfillment in helping other people. She talked about her father who never allowed her to give in or give up. And she talked about her rock, her mainstay, her husband, and how he was always there for her in his strong, gentle way, his warm hand reaching through the bars of the hospital bed, flowing strength into her when she first regained consciousness after surgery, giving her the will to live, loving her with her scars, tubes, bags, bottles, and all, the long telephone calls in the middle of the night from the cabin in New Jersey to her hospital bed in Philadelphia when the pain was so bad that she couldn't sleep and needed help just getting through one more night, her silent Santa who was the workhorse of Christmas Express, her Captain when they were sailing, and always the wind beneath her wings. She talked about her deep and abiding faith in God being the cornerstone of her recovery, giving her strength when the pain was more than she could bear and keeping her believing that after the darkness there would be light. She quoted her favorite scripture from the Bible, "They that wait upon the Lord shall renew their strength: They shall mount up with wings as eagles: They shall run, and not be weary: And they shall walk and not faint." And she talked about the actual Great Comebacks Award, which is a crystal eagle perched on a crystal ball and ironically how the eagle, representing courage and determination, had always been her symbol and held a personal meaning for her. She often looked at Glenn and other faces in the room when she spoke. Her words created tremendous emotion, and everyone was moved to tears. She ended by saying, "If there is one thing I want to leave you with, it's a message of hope, of hope for the future. The next time you or someone you love is facing depression or is discouraged, remember me, the woman who mounted the wings of an eagle and flew into an untroubled sky."

For a few seconds there remained complete silence. Then there was thundering applause as everyone, all 600 people, rose to their feet, clapping wildly and wiping their eyes.

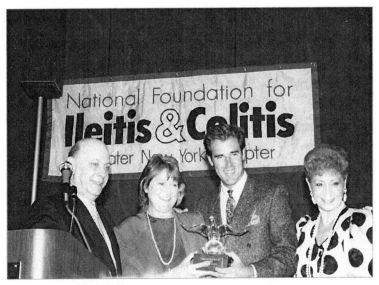

Annie accepting the Great Comebacks Award from Rolf Benirschke

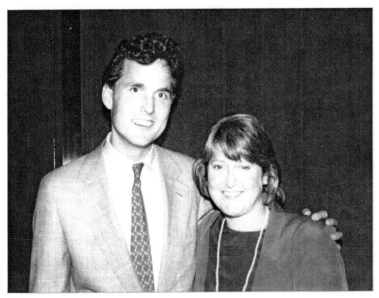

Annie pictured with Marvin Bush, son of President George Bush

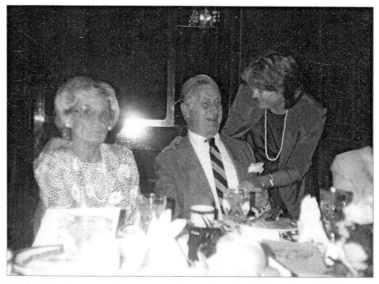

Annie, after her acceptance speech, greeting her father where he is sitting with his wife, Bobbie

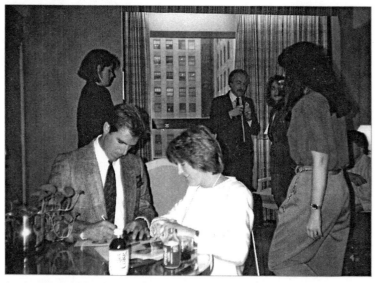

Annie with Rolf Benirschke before interviews

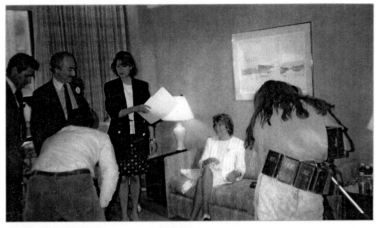

Annie with photographers and people associated with the award

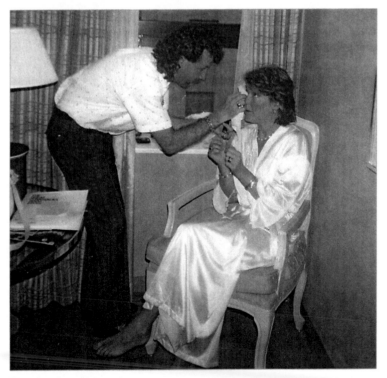

The glamour treatment

CHAPTER TWELVE

Death Has No Identity

❧

AFTER ANNIE AND GLENN returned from New York, ConvaTec followed up the grand weekend of events by sending a photographer to Cape May Court House in order to capture some more shots of their new "star." This is the letter written by the photographer after that shoot:

Dear Sailors,

I just wanted to drop a note to express my thanks for the wonderful time we all enjoyed with you at our recent Great Comebacks photoshoot. It was terrific to be out on the ocean with two experienced sea hands like yourselves, even if I did turn green once I went below deck. And I enjoyed seeing the handiwork in your home and spending time with the animals (at least those that didn't scratch or bite).

Your courage, steadfastness, and love are an inspira-
tion to witness. In an era in which people are consumed
with things rather than relationships, your faith in and
dedication to each other offers a refreshing contrast.

I hope we have a chance to work on another project
in the future. If you are passing through Princeton, be
sure to stop in to see us.

> *Sincerely,*
> *Allen Owen*

Allen's reference to Glenn and the devotion that Annie and Glenn shared is no surprise. They were a team and continued to be as one until the very end.

After Annie ruptured her Achilles tendons, Glenn started plans to have a heated pool, both for therapy and enjoyment.

An above ground pool is much less costly than an in-ground pool but not as attractive or easily accessible. Glenn came up with a compromise. He dug down several feet in the place where they planned to have the pool, and raised the surrounding area with the dirt taken from the hole, grading it downward toward the house. An above ground pool, four-feet deep, was placed into the hole and Glenn constructed an extensive slatted wood deck that surrounded it. He then added a wheelchair accessible walkway between it and the house.

Many happy and restful times were spent in the pool and poolside, and when family and friends came to visit, it was great entertainment for adults and children alike.

Even early in their marriage, Annie had to spend extended times in bed before and after her surgeries. Glenn wanted her to be able to be on the first floor, so he built an addition that looked and functioned like a family room, but had a bed. It was a spacious room with three walls of windows giving her the next best thing to being outside. It was wonderful to still be able to experience nature without actually having to be outside.

The view from her bed and patio looked out over the pond where Hooter, the Canadian goose, resided. Hooter had come to them with an injured wing that left him unable to fly, so the pond at Nature's Way became his permanent home. Seasonally, other geese would keep him company while migrating and stay a while before moving on. Other inhabitants of the pond were a few otters and turtles. Through the years, other geese, swans, and ducks made their home at Nature's Way.

For Annie's viewing pleasure, many different birds were attracted to the abundant and strategically placed feeders and birdhouses. One of their cats could usually be spotted perusing the territory, and their dogs had a great time charging a few feet into the water, barking at turtles.

Annie would rejoice when the first signs of spring appeared, with early flowers coming to life and trees with tiny green leaves looking like lace against a sky blue background. With the arrival of spring, Annie was rejuvenated by the new life that was emerging all around her, and as always, it gave her new hope. As it is exhilarating to experience spring after a long winter, so is it gratefully appreciated to feel well after months of recovery from serious pain and illness.

In the summer there was an abundance and variety of multiple shades of green with colorful flowers planted to accent nature's own contributions.

Fall brought a myriad of bountiful colors as the woodland trees daily increased their intensity until there was a palette of vibrant colors surrounding the cabin.

In winter, snow provided beauty and peacefulness with snow-laden branches and animal tracks that appeared in an otherwise undisturbed carpet of white. There were also plenty of dreary, snowless winter days where bare branches were etched against a gray sky.

Just as the decades of seasons came and went, so did Annie's health, and in the last year of her life, she was mostly confined to her bed and wheelchair.

As much as I appreciate being able to enjoy nature from my bed in the addition, I am getting claustrophobic and longing for an open sky and sparkling vista of the sea. Oh God, how I long for being "on the hook" or a lazy motor sail to our mooring down the channel after hours on the ocean with the ruby sun setting behind the Lobster House Schooner, standing on the bow-sprit, arms around the forestay, jib furled, boom mewing with the swaying rhythm of Freyja. Sometimes, if we hadn't set sail, we would dink to the Lobster House for fresh fish on the barby or pack up a cooler of munchies and take a lazy meander through the lush green marshes.

Egrets' bellies were pink in the sunset's glow, with dark water curving in and out, mirror still, save the tinkling droplets from baitfish.

It hurts, yet is comforting, to write memories of yesterdays while visualizing the places, hearing the sounds, seeing the colors, smelling comforting fragrances, touching the earth with its gritty, cool sand, moist dirt, and dry leaves of the woods. I breathe in the sweet, salty scent of the beach and fresh tang of the bay breeze, hear the sea gulls laughing overhead, the bark of a great blue heron as he glides effortlessly along the shoreline and the familiar mew of an osprey. The wind is rustling in the treetops, the blue green of the ocean is breaking into white crested waves with bubbling foam popping at the water's edge as tiny pipers skitter just out of reach, their matchstick legs a blur of motion. Cool, wet, dark sand pulls at my feet as the tide rushes back to the bosom of its being. The water's sun-sequined surface is gaily calling me to immerse myself in her cold, wet embrace, then a wave is breaking over me causing a spontaneous somersault; salt water goes up my nose, and I wipe it away as inconspicuously as possible.

Then I'm galumphing through the shallow waves, heading for my chair where my towel, book, and lotion are waiting. After a brisk rub with the towel and laying it carefully over the chair, I get my book, visor, sunglasses, and suntan lotion out of the beach bag. Patiently I apply the suntan lotion, being especially careful not to get sand mixed in or it feels like greasy sandpaper. Then it is time to plop into the chair, scoot around a bit to face the sun in the best possible direction, and with the visor on to curb the reflection, I settle into a good ol' fat novel.

I can hear, smell, and feel it all as I lie in bed. It is another brilliant, sun-drenched day. Paralyzing back and leg pain again has rendered me in couch- or bed-potato status. Percocet and levo have an annoying side effect of lethargy.

I write for someone to talk to, to express what is within me. My journal never judges me, no Pollyanna, I can fight one more round with drivel. I exist on memories of times past. Oddly, rarely, very rarely do I think about so many years of multiple surgeries, being away from Glenn and my home, my critters, missing life, weddings, family and birthday celebrations. The only graduation I have ever attended was from high school. My AA, BA, and M.Ed. degrees were all mailed to me. I was just shy of getting my Ph.D.

I like to remember our many special happy moments cruising on the Chesapeake, three trips to the Virgin Islands or on the hook anywhere, taking care of our "rehab" critters, opossums, skunks, birds of prey, squirrels, song birds, turtles, geese, swans, and of course raccoons, my precious special ones. For the first time in thirty years, I had to let go a hungry, ill wee baby coon who came to me. His mom had abandoned him because of "natural selection." This little runt cried for my help, wild and unafraid. You see I was totally physically unable to reach down and pick up this little helpless critter, and I watched with tears and a broken heart as she limped away.

When Annie was confined to her bed in the addition, pain often denied her sleep at night and she would watch endless hours of classic movies on TV. It used to be that when she was well enough she would rejoice in returning to their bed upstairs where Glenn's warm body welcomed her. Sadly, that way of life was now over.

Annie had always had a great zest for life and lived it to the fullest whenever she was healthy. She was bound and determined to make up for the lost time she had missed being ill. After regaining her health, Annie would go full tilt ahead, relishing every moment of the day. There was so much living to catch up on: animal care, sailing odysseys, long walks in the woods, birding, gardening, Christmas Express and other volunteer work that fed her soul, friends to connect with, projects to work on, the crafts that she always wanting to expand . . . whatever she did, she did with great enthusiasm and joy. Oh, to feel well, what a blessing and one she never took for granted. But now she no longer could look forward to healthy and happy times because she was trapped in a body that had reached the point of no return.

It was heartbreaking for Annie to have to let go of the life that she had been living, and giving up her beloved Christmas Express was one of the most difficult. Even in the last few years that Annie ran Christmas Express, the dedicated effort that she put into it was taking an increasingly devastating toll on her body.

The time came when Annie was no longer capable of doing the shopping for Christmas Express. So she said good-bye to the marathon shopping that had been part of the adventure each year.

"Oh, it was great fun," she told me, "because you're not spending your own money and you know every cent is going to help people."

She laughed when she told the story about the Christmas when she was unable to walk because of a broken foot, so a friend pushed her up and down the aisles of a store on a huge warehouse cart. There was Annie sitting in the middle of this large, flat cart surrounded by books and toys and clothes piled high. It was so typical of Annie. She never shied away from anything because of her health. If there was a way to get something done, she would go for it, and it was always a memorable experience full of wonderful laughter. As she suffered pain and fatigue, she found comfort in warm memories of the love that she felt from being instrumental in making so many people's lives happier, and she expressed those thoughts through her carefully handwritten thank-you notes.

There was a year when Annie was consigned to running Christmas Express by remote control from a bed at the University of Pennsylvania Hospital, where she had been a patient since late September. In a telephone interview Annie said:

"I'm stuck up here and can't do what I normally would, so it's all falling on Glenn. He's the head elf this year. I've made a list of suggestions of what to buy. I'm going to be home in time for Christmas if I have to drag these pumps with me." Then, referring to all of the machines she was hooked up to at the hospital, she added, "I look a little bit like a Christmas tree myself—I'll just put a bow on my head and I will be Glenn's tree!"

As Annie became more housebound, she became more limited in what she could do to help.

"I can only do it with my voice," she told the reporter of a local newspaper in the final year she would see Christmas Express in action. "My mouth and my heart still work but my body parts are giving up. I know that Christmas Express will continue if I can find someone to pass my work on to as one passes on the light from a candle. It all started with one candle lit by seeing a very real need right here in our very own backyard; I remember back sixteen years ago to when I first tutored that pregnant thirteen-year-old girl. One candle lit another and another until it just encircled our county."

Annie talks about a Christmas that lead up to her having to give up her charity.

I had been getting progressively sicker and was desperately trying to hang on for Christmas at the cabin. The alternative was too horrible to contemplate. But alas, the "bod" won out. I fully obstructed on Christmas Eve day. Glenn played ambulance driver yet again and zoomed me up to HUP while at times leaning out the window, yelling, "Medical emergency!" as he demonstrated his race driver skills. Once we reached the emergency entrance a policeman stopped us for speeding and an illegal turn to which I responded rather graphically by throwing up on his shiny shoes. *Realizing the seriousness of the situation, he hastily signaled us forward.*

Tearfully we had a heart-wrenching good-bye in a gray, empty hospital room. Choking back tears with a rather shaky but determined smile, I said, "I'll see you tomorrow, Lovie. We will be each other's Christmas. I'll get a double of Demerol to celebrate...."

He was leaving to go home to an empty cabin on Christmas Eve. It was all just too awful and I thought I would burst with sadness for him.

After he left I allowed myself to dissolve into tears, and then within a few minutes I heard foot-steps coming down the hall and looking up through my tears there was Glenn filling the doorframe. His eyes were twinkling as he said, "I forgot something..." and he carefully pulled a beautiful Santa from behind his back. "I thought you might need a buddy." My tears became sobs as I pulled the red velvet body toward me. When I gained some composure, I looked at the Santa, marveling over his gaily smiling face that was intricately painted on fine porcelain. I touched each little toy in his sack, so adorable, and then stroked his soft, fluffy beard. "Oh. Glenn, how...? Where...? When...?"

He answered with, "I figured that you might not be able to be home for Christmas so I went to the gift gallery last week."

I held onto that Santa throughout the night,
warmed and comforted by the love that brought
him to me.

I have embraced the memory of that special
Christmas, knowing that our greatest gift was the
love and sacrifice of our Christ, exemplified again
and again by that precious Hippie who figured I
needed something to hug.

Back at home after she left one of her innumerable hospital stays, Annie would often need to be bedridden for months at a time. It was then that all of the work that she had put into Nature's Way came back to her; for every bit of love that Annie and Glenn gave their animals, their love was returned in equal amounts. Animals instinctively know when you are not well and will stay by your side with undivided loyalty. When Annie was in bed, it wasn't unusual to have her body lined with several critters of various species. Annie could feel the warmth of each furry creature snuggled close against her and would be comforted by their presence and the softness of their fur and beautiful faces.

Looking from her bed to the right and front of the cabin, she could see a visitor walking up the brick path from the parking area, or Glenn coming in from his shop to check on her. In front of her was a wide view of the woods, and to her left, sliding glass doors led out to a small patio and Gramma's chaise lounge, which held so many loving memories from her childhood. When Annie was recuperating from surgery and the weather was accommodating, she could leave her bed to lie on the chaise. Beyond the patio was the pond, a little bridge, and a waterfall.

Many times throughout her life I had seen Annie very sick, but one of her worst times was when, in addition to constant pain, she had frequent spasms of excruciating pain that shot through her in spite of the additional pain meds that Glenn slipped to her when she was in the hospital. Annie had multiple hairline fractures in her back from so many years of steroids causing severe osteoporosis that was in addition to the ubiquitous pain in her gut. At times the pain was so intense it was difficult for her to breathe.

> *Pain is worsening daily; familiar intensity is a burning reminder of what I try most to forget. Dr. Peter's prognosis tearfully given, instinctively denied by me, now echoes strongly like knocks on the final door down the hall of hope.*
>
> *"Your gut is closing down, Anne, no more can be done. Edema is in your intestine, and it will eventually weaken to the point of perforation. You will have to be on permanent hyperalimentation. No, you will never eat again. We may find a site in your groin; the head vascular surgeon at Hopkins may try. Your history of sepsis is a real deterrent and threatens the reality of this port placement."*
>
> *So it is hyperalimentation or die—before the summer? Oh Lord, what lies ahead this year?*
>
> *Writing is my way of presenting reality. Once a thought or feeling is put into words and expressed on paper, it becomes more real.*

The pain is all too real. I tried, I tried so hard this past weekend. It was spring, what should have been a beautiful, breezy boat time, but I was not able to walk upright. It is unfair to put so much of a burden on Glenn.

I don't think I am scared of what may or may not be happening. I am extremely ashamed, however, that I didn't do more with the past two years that God blessed me with, years of comparative health. I felt sincerely that I had been healed. There was no medical explanation for my ability to eat, to absorb nutrition. The endoscopic showed beyond a doubt that my intestines were strictured by extrinsic adhesions narrowing to less than the circumference of the inside cylinder of a Bic pen.

So now, now in a frenzied attempt to get it all in, I ask a friend to take me to the beach with internal tears and fears spilling over into my mother ocean. Comforted again by my friend and the beach I think, Maybe it isn't too late. Maybe if I really take it easy with a limited diet, rest, up the steroids, maybe I can quell this flare-up. Please, Lord, may I have some more time? Time to put my home in order. Time to write overdue letters of gratitude and love. How do I clear my desk? How do I prepare now for what seems to be inevitable? Is it inevitable? Dear Lord, can there be one more miracle—I am not ready yet.

Well, it seems that God was listening because without explanation, which totally baffled the doctors, Annie was able to continue eating and recovered to live many more years. But with the years of abuse that her body had taken, the time finally came when it was no longer possible to rise again for one more miracle.

> *Death has no identity, being, or reason of its own. There is no measure of completion. Just as you can't be a little bit pregnant. I thought you couldn't be a little bit dead, or can you? I have lived through code blue and a seven-week coma. There is a nonretractable component in human nature that renders it absolutely impossible for us to face or accept our own mortality. Vulnerability lies as an open wound. Until recently death was just a word or a diagnosis, a challenge rather than an ending. Death is an abstract concept and I am unable to truly embrace the whole concept of my life being over, kaput. Death and dying has a face now, a reality heretofore veiled.*

On an early August morning in 2008, Annie was rushed to the hospital by ambulance after several days of being very sick with food poisoning, which caused severe dehydration and then seizures. The next day she crashed with heart failure, and Glenn was asked if they should bring her back or let her go. Without hesitation Glenn said to bring her back. Her kidneys shut down but then showed signs of improving. It was her white count that was threatening with a count of 30,000 compared to the normal rate, which is around 7,000-10,000. If the count hadn't come down, her respiratory could have suffered to such a degree that her emphysema would have done her in.

In a letter to my close friend Julie, I confided, "I wonder if I should be resigned to her going? Annie has suffered so incredibly for most of her life and her body is in such deplorable shape that part of me would hate to see her having to face more pain. I think maybe we want her to survive for all of us who love her so much and not for her quality of life. It is possible that she may recover simply because she has beaten the odds so many times before but I really think that this time it is different and it may be time to let go."

It is hard not to love Annie. The nurses at the hospital are really caring and attentive; Annie quickly made an impact on their lives with her indomitable spirit and humor. Knowing that Annie was always thrilled with furry visitors that melted her heart, I brought in an unusually calm, adorable Schnoodle puppy (miniature Schnauzer/poodle mix) who lay quietly on her bed with his head resting on Annie. Annie was delighted with her sweet little visitor, and she tried to hide the puppy among her stuffed animals when one of the nurses came in. The nurse just looked at her and with a smile said, "Don't bother, honey, we know the puppy is here."

Annie's eating was becoming very sporadic but she asked for some unusual foods such as pickles, sweet gherkins, and some dill wedges along with sauerkraut. We were all too willing to give her anything she wanted. Around 11:30 a.m. one day, when her half-brother, Phil, was visiting her, Annie's lunch was delivered, and when Annie lifted the lid on the "gourmet" surprise that awaited her, she quickly said, "It's this shit that's going to kill me!" They both laughed. Phil asked her what she'd like to have and without much hesitation, she said, "I want a Whopper!" So off to Burger King he went for that with some fries and a fresh Dr. Pepper. She tore into that stuff right away and loved every bite of it. Next time she said she wanted the same thing but with a black-and-white milk shake, and oh, yes, no tomatoes on the burger, please.

Throughout their marriage, Annie endured many long, painful, and sleepless days and nights. Many of these were in the hospital, away from Glenn, where she could be for months at a time. One of her writings talked about these tough times.

> *Things are getting pretty tough emotionally in the ICU. God, I hate to be apart from Glenn. Thoughts and words unspoken echo in my head. Without him to speak with, touch, hug, I feel like I'm only wearing one shoe. He punctuates my days with exclamation marks, exclaiming my blessings with simple caring gestures. I love him so that it hurts sometimes. When we are apart and I get a notion of what life would be like without my partner, waves of anxiety and fear ripple through me. Glenn is the center of my being. I breathe because he is my air.*
>
> *Over all the years of pictures of us together, there is not one where we aren't touching: a hug, holding hands, Glenn's arm around my shoulder, or*

*my arm through his or sitting in his lap. That physi-
cal touching ends at the last minute before one of
my God-knows-how-many surgeries and resumes
the minute we are allowed to see each other again.*

*I've always said that following surgery, there
are two kinds of hugs. Hug #1 is sitting down or
half down in bed. This is an upper-body hug with
Glenn leaning down or over to me. One hand usually planted firmly on the couch or bed. His arm
stiff—elbow locked to bear the weight for both of
us as I lean forward, arms outstretched, feeling
the warmth of Glenn enfolding me with the scent
of cedar, sweat, or salt marsh—comforting and
familiar. Always ending with a sloppy or sweet—
depending on his mood—kiss on the forehead—a
warm spot that will stay with me all day.*

*Hug #2 is a recovery benchmark after months
of Hug #1. When I can finally stand—term used
loosely as sometimes I cheat, holding on to the bed
or pump stand or both but in upright posture—then
I can enjoy a full-body press! Glenn, my tree, is now
more tentative, finding the place tenderly where he
can safely put his hands and arms without eliciting
an "ow" or sucked-in breath from me. Position and
height-/weight-bearing ability established, he smiles
and I giggle. Face accentuated with my signature
raccoon eyes, literally my head would be resting
anywhere from his belly, midsternum, depending
on my degree of position, to absolute joy, that warm,
sweet, oh-so-familiar hollow where his neck joins*

his shoulder. Full-body hug—then I am home in the
safe, healing harbor of my lover's arms.
   So, a full-body hug has a long symbolic history
with us. And boy do I need one now! Credo born:
I reach for my love saying, HUG FULL LENGTH
GIVES US STRENGTH. He half-smiles, and for
that quiet moment we are safe in each other's arms.

As Annie's health became increasingly dire, I wrote
to Julie of Annie's condition. "Annie is in a difficult place
right now, not knowing whether to live a little longer or die
sooner. She is getting ready to go but can't bear the thought
of not seeing Glenn's face ever again or being with the rest
of the ones she loves. It will play out in time and we will
all miss her terribly and realize that we have known an
extraordinary person.

"She is getting weaker and thinner by the day. Her
cheeks aren't near as full as before and her hands are nothing but skin and bone. I just can't see it being more than a
few weeks now before she departs this life here on earth
but it wouldn't surprise me for her to surprise me. She is
still with us, but it is just a matter of time now because she
is off of all medical help and just getting pain management.

"Lynnie went down to see Annie and stayed there all
day. She said that Annie was being Annie and cracking
jokes so the plan of her going to say good-bye didn't feel
like good-bye at all.

"Ray and I are going to see her on Saturday, and I
don't know if that will be for the last time or not. I prefer
to think that it will not be the last time even if it is because

I can't imagine walking out the door knowing that I will never see her again or tell her I love her one more time. Her theme song has always been 'Stayin' Alive,' but now I think it has switched to 'I'm coming home, I've done my time.' I think emotionally she is just about ready to accept it.

"I'm quite sure that it is the news of not being able to ever go home to the cabin and her critters again that has made the difference. When Glenn had to tell her that she was never going home again, he was sobbing. We all know that this is for the best and that this time is the right time, but that doesn't seem to make it any easier. The doctors have taken any decision making away from Glenn. He is no longer physically or emotionally capable of the twenty-four-hour care that Annie needs.

"At this point I strangely feel more resolved to the situation. I have accepted that this time she may live a little longer, but I don't think she will ever have any quality of life again and that means that she would probably be better off "going home" as she puts it, and she doesn't mean to the cabin.

"She was asleep when Ray and I arrived. She awoke quickly. Annie looked up at me and asked, 'Is this the day?' I told her that it was in God's hands. I see her struggling with that decision as though it were hers to make. She says, 'I don't know what God wants me to do.' I told her that he would let her know when the time comes.

"I don't think she's fighting to live any longer. In fact, I believe she is truly ready and willing to make her final journey. Her body is so used to fighting that it hasn't recognized what her mind wants to do. Oh yes, she is afraid. But not of dying. She's afraid of not seeing Glenn, her critters, and her family anymore. I told her we would always see her in our memories and that she'll always be with us in our hearts."

Once Annie gave the directive to not receive any more medical assistance, I knew that there were probably only a few months left. It was late August and with time running out, every few days I would drive a four-hour round trip to see Annie at the hospital and then go to the cabin where Glenn and I would sit and talk on the side of the pool with our legs dangling in the water while I recorded amazing stories of Annie and their lives together that were filled with joy, thrills, agony, commitment, and fun.

Glenn draws out his words in a very relaxed way and always holds the moment before he speaks to think about what he is going to say. He laughs easily when thinking about the fun he had with Annie, and it was a very special time for me being with just him.

So many years and so much life have passed since we first got to know each other. Glenn's hair, which was once red, wavy, and past his shoulders, is now shorter and has turned gray, and he has long since shaved off his famous beard. We talked about the animals and Annie and how he was dealing with a life so different than he had expected. He said that when they got married he told Annie, referring to her health, that they would just take one step at a time and would handle whatever came their way. Neither one anticipated the extent and severity of her illness and complications.

One of the things we talked about was the time when Annie was at Ithaca College and was briefly engaged until her fiancé with the advice of his father, a doctor, broke it off after her first surgery. Glenn couldn't fathom how someone who was in love with Annie could walk away and abandon her because of an unsure future. Glenn loved Annie, and her illness didn't scare him off. He loved Annie with a complete acceptance that few people would be capable of given her illness. He was willing to be there for her and with her through whatever future they would face together. They had far from a normal life together, and although there were exceptionally bad times, there were also many exceptionally good times. God just may have had something to do with bringing Glenn into Annie's life.

It was at this time that Glenn also told me about all of the journals Annie had been keeping throughout the years. I had no idea that she had done such extensive writing in so many journals. She never talked about them. I knew that Annie wrote beautifully because of the many letters that she had written to me throughout the years, but the journals were a wonderful surprise, and I was delighted to see the extent of what she had documented and the care with which she crafted her words. With so much of her life being told by her in her own written word, there were great stories, and I loved that she also expressed many of her profound personal insights.

A thought just grazed on the meadow of my horizonless mind. During our youth to midtwenties, our time is spent with school and accomplishing goals. Our expectations and our achievements are only limited by our desire, boundless hope, energy, and fascination with new discoveries. Each day, each hour, and every moment come feelings never to be experienced again.

When I was younger, healthier, and more enthusiastic, I learned more, reached for more, and achieved more. But goals like graduating from increasingly higher levels of education or getting jobs were not the end in themselves. They were for the triumph, the feeling of worth that emerged from the process and the struggles. I felt fulfilled by the desire to become, the desire to be. The forward momentum, the mental and physical motion, propelled me into my days.

Today after mind-wracking pain subsided to a manageable level I allowed myself a few hours of numb free fall into an abyss of utter despair. This half-life I have called mine walks the precarious line between use and usefulness. Success is a relative concept.

I unearthed two boxes full of journals, written during trips on Freyja, and flipped through a few pages. Some were stuck together with ink smears. The year wasn't important. Beauty surrounded us along with the unfettered joy at just plain being aboard. Images came smiling back; I was so caught up in the blessing of the moment. I could visualize images of dawn, blissful sail smackin' romps up the bay, dinners under the stars, gunkholing, or "What's around that spit?" With adrenaline-pumping squalls and a myriad of sights, sounds, smells, and feelings,

*it was all a multihued, multiremembered, richly
textured tapestry of odysseys on* Freyja.

    In *my glass-half-empty mode, I thought,* Gad,
what a waste of space and time my life has
become. *But as I write, I know the glass is half full,
running over actually, filled with the love and care
of Glenn, a home built and filled with his talent
and creative genius . . . .*

The following is the last letter that Annie ever wrote
to her beloved Glenn, sometime before she was hospitalized for the last time.

*Hi cute Hippie of mine. It is 2:30 a.m. Sometimes the
first thing I see when I awake, as my eyes grudgingly
open and my focus sharpens, is a large bright scarlet-pink
hibiscus you picked for me and placed in a tall glass on
my end table. Or it could be a lovely piece of sunshine
with wee yellow wild flowers in a small antique bottle.
They are another sweet reminder of the grace of another
day with you by my side.*

    *Pain is usually my first waking awareness, but it's
bumped aside with the welcome sensation of warmth
and worth. "He loves me still." The color of your caring
is ever changing with the flowers that awaken my soul.*

    *Sometimes it is an e-mail you have printed late
at night while I'm once again unconsciously sleeping. It is a sweet something to wake up to, and I feel
a rush of tenderness and gratitude for you and your
thoughtfulness. For the millionth time, I feel so very*

lucky and blessed for having you as my partner in this roller-coaster ride we deem life. I thank God every day for the sheer blessing of you in my life. Is it possible to love you more after so many years? Yep, it is! I still well up with tears many times when you come into a room, just plain looking at my handsome partner whose talent and intelligence is matched only by his honor and compassion. You are my forever hero. How lucky I am to have a man like you, supporting and encouraging me with never a burst of temper or impatience. How gentle and caring you are and always my advocate, never letting the doctors get away with anything. With you in my life, my wish to live was always stronger than my will to die.

This last siege of body malfunctions has been the worst scenario that we have ever experienced. The routine recovery from so many surgeries seems like a walk in the park compared to this horror. Recovery always involved the healing power of being aboard Freyja. *There were excited butterflies as we prepared for a cruise on the Chesapeake, the sparkling mother ocean, cool breezes, the snap of sails catching the cooling wind, your ubiquitous sailing smile while straddling the helm, spacing out under open skies, gunkholing, walking through the woods with leaves crunching beneath our every footfall, finding familiar beloved anchorages, swaying gently on the hook, doing our thing, you eternally futzing, me in my spot reading, writing with my mug of tea or Dr. Pepper, and Tippy at my side, at peace with each other and the inspiring beauty around us.*

Honestly, Hippie, my love for you has literally kept me alive. But, darling, the past too many months, with you having to do everything for me, the house, the critters, never having time for yourself and never, never complaining . . . You deserve so much more my precious husband—laughter, sailing!!—a wife that can help you like a wife should.

I have watched you day after day after day, cooking, vacuuming, running errands for my meds, and all the time my heart is aching while my body is yearning to be useful, helpful.

Remember yesterday when I told you the turning point? I have now reached the stage of indifference. You know the stages of facing death, our own or of one much loved; denial, guilt, anger, grief, and finally acceptance. I have been trapped so long, so too long in this body that is no longer mine. When you lose your freedom so completely, when you compound this loss by robbing the one you love of his freedom, it is intolerable.

Remember our wedding vows so deliberately and joyously written as we raced to the rehearsal in your Mustang? We said, through tears and with trembling, unsteady voices: "I choose you to be my husband/wife."

Oh, Hippie mine, the sheer joy of that day. We would never be apart again. The dreams we shared with our whole life ahead of us.

Oh yeah, we knew that I wouldn't be healthy, but oh my, we surely had no idea of the hospital horrors that awaited, the agonizing months and months of loneliness, pain, and uncertainty while desperately missing each other.

I learned to swallow my tears, assume a hopeful, even happy countenance. I had to be patient, for grief and worry only worsened the pain and surely never helped recovery.

Oh, how I lived for weekends, your strong warm gentle hug, your dancing green eyes, the smell of you, cedar dust and baby shampoo.

Then, my darling, I was struggling to come home, home to you, home to my critters, my cabin, my pond, trees and shrubs, and the rumble of the bay with each undulation of the tide admonishing me for abandoning her while wet and gruffly welcoming me home.

Whenever I feel too unbearably sad, I close my eyes and feel, no re-feel your warm, firm good-morning kiss before you left me for the day.

You looked into my eyes, your green eyes twinkling and a slight smile played upon your lips.

You held my gaze briefly, wanting to be sure that I knew you loved me.

Then you kissed me ever so sweetly, not a peck given absentmindedly, but a kiss.

I can still feel your arms around me, gently hugging. One final look into my eyes and then you were gone. Can you please hold that last kiss for the rest of a lifetime?

Annie passed away peacefully on the morning of December 9, 2008, at 6:50. She wasn't alone. A nurse's aide was with her reading to her from Gramma's Bible. Glenn had been called and he rushed to the hospital. He went to her side and took her hand. Annie's eyes met his, there was a faint smile, and then she was gone. It is as if she waited for him to be with her and have his face be the last thing she saw before her eyes closed forever.

Many members of her family drove from a distance and arrived early at Annie's "celebration of life" service on Saturday, December 20, in Cape May Court House. Glenn had requested that we wear colors rather than black because Annie disliked black attire at funerals.

As we entered the room, we immediately saw five large three-by-four-foot picture boards placed on easels at the front of the room. Every board had a different theme and was covered with pictures of her life's journey. A neighbor and good friend, Audrey, did a very dedicated and amazing job creating them. This tribute to Annie was very emotional. I felt like she was in the room with us. Friends and family went from board to board crying and laughing through their tears. You could see people pointing as they found themselves in a picture, remembering a special time, but then all times with Annie were special.

As more family members arrived, we hugged and sometimes sobbed in each other's arms. Finally we were requested to sit for the ceremony.

To begin the celebration, Annie's cousin Stephen walked down the aisle playing "Amazing Grace" and "Coming Home" on the bagpipes.

Among other contributions from family, Annie's favorite passage was read, Isaiah 40:28–31:

Have you not known?
Have you not heard?

The Everlasting God, the Lord,
The Creator of the ends of the earth,
Neither faints nor is weary.
His understanding is unsearchable.
He gives power to the weak,
And to those who have no might He increases strength.
Even the youths shall faint and be weary,
And the young men shall utterly fall,
But those who wait on the Lord
Shall renew their strength;
They shall mount up with wings like eagles,
They shall run and not be weary,
They shall walk and not faint.

Lowrey gave the eulogy, which was touching and tearful.

Following the eulogy, my son David read the lyrics to a song he had written for Annie some years ago. It has a beautiful melody with loving lyrics that he sings with his guitar, but he chose to just read the lyrics because he was too emotional to sing.

The pastor, Dr. Frank Reeder, and Annie had been closely connected. He knew Annie very well as they had enjoyed many a discussion about God, heaven, and the scriptures over a dozen or more years. He smiled when he said that her language was at times a bit salty, but quickly added that when she slipped and let out an occasional expletive that it didn't make her spirit or her faith any less wonderful. We all laughed because we knew

Annie. The pastor was wonderful and spoke from a deep knowledge and understanding of Annie. He sang two of her favorite songs.

An adjoining room was opened up to accommodate the larger-than-expected crowd that was there to celebrate Annie's life. An abundance of programs had been printed but no one had anticipated the number of people that would come to say good-bye, and they ran out but promised to send one if requested.

When asked who all those people were, other than family and friends, Glenn said in his quiet way, some were people he worked with and others were just some of the many people Annie had helped or had touched along the way. They had come to pay their last respects.

The reception at the Avalon Golf Club was generously given by Annie's sister, Tyler.

It had been brought to Glenn's attention that it is illegal to spread ashes in the water at Stone Harbor Point, which had been Annie's wish, so Glenn went at midnight in the cloak of darkness to carry out Annie's request.

Annie and Glenn would have been married thirty-two years the next month on the seventeenth of January.

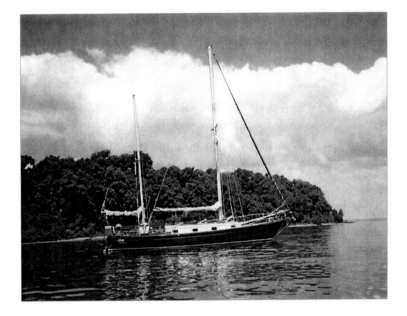

Love Always Annie

Annie, you're sailing away
To your own special island.
The days are long
And the nights are longer.
When it comes to life,
There is no one stronger.

    The sea gets rough
    And the tides they rise.
    But you are tough,
    there is no compromise.
    Love always, Annie.

With the wind behind your back
You've got the courage you've always had.
There are not words enough to say,
The times sailing the ocean and the bay.
Live for tomorrow,
Love for today,
Love always, Annie.

> The sea gets rough
> And the tides they rise,
> But you are tough,
> There is no compromise.
> Love always, Annie.

—David Heaver

CHAPTER THIRTEEN

The Glorious Gift of a Morning

"What sheer joy there is in just plain living and allowing time to become a friend instead of an adversary."

—ANNIE

⁂

THROUGHOUT THE PROCESS of compiling this story of Annie's life, I felt her presence emanate from the pages of her journals and also from the way that our entwined lives came together in the structure of this book. I felt Annie tugging at me not to end with her death. It was as if she was saying in her soft voice, "Remember, Sweetie"—she would call me affectionate names—"remember how I ended my Great Comebacks Award speech?" She had said, "If there is one thing I want to leave you with, it's a message of hope, of hope for the future . . . the woman who mounted the wings of an eagle and flew into an untroubled sky."

I remember, Annie, and I know all of those whose lives you touched remember too. That is how we should best remember you.

What a glorious gift of a morning! I'm up with the sun. She is peeking in the companionway, scolding me for missing her golden entrance over the horizon. "I was waiting for you to warm things up a bit," I muttered as I reluctantly left my snug berth.

The early morning chill sent me scurrying forward to turn on the stove. Hopping on one leg, I struggled into my pants with the frosty air nipping at my bottom and I again questioned our sanity.

With coffee and cocoa on and wearing three layers of shirts and sweats, I climbed topside. Geese were flying overhead honking good morning. Ospreys were mewing and gliding nearby searching for breakfast. The sky was a brilliant deep blue with just a few wisps of cotton clouds and the sun, which had made a sparkling path to our stern, was warming me.

I saw three, no four, ospreys circling over my shoulder and then my heart jumped; one was too large to be a fish hawk. Grabbing the binoculars, I held my breath in anticipation. Yep, it was an eagle. His golden talons were accentuated as he swooped in and landed in a nearby tree. I could tell that he was an adolescent because his head was still brown.

What a treat! He stayed for quite a while surveying our little cove. I kept the binoculars glued on him, and every so often he would turn toward me and I could see his yellow beak and piercing yellow eyes. "What do you see up there, you grand creature?" Then leaning his head forward, he took off, and with one flap of those powerful wings, he was airborne, gliding over the meadow and beyond the trees. What a way to start the day!

I love all of Annie's eagle stories, from her sighting them in the wild to the eagle being the symbol for her Great Comebacks Award and for the reference of the eagle in her favorite passage from the Bible that was read at her celebration of life ceremony. "But those who wait on the Lord shall renew their strength; They shall mount up with wings like eagles, they shall run and not be weary, they shall walk and not faint." The eagle always represented the strength and courage that Annie lived by. A dear lifelong friend of hers wrote a letter after Annie's death, and after quoting the passage she said, "Can't you just see her now? Fly, Annie, fly." Those words brought me to tears because of the thought of Annie flying with her eagles and being free of earthly pain.

Annie contended with incredible challenges through a simple love of life and seeking joy and freedom from pain in whatever measure each day. One way she achieved this was through gunkholing. Gunkholing is a term used for meandering around the little coves and inlets of the shoreline in a small boat. It was during these expeditions that she experienced her greatest taste of freedom from the physical limitations that plagued her for so many months out of every given year.

Oh, Oh!! Glenn gave me my birthday present early, a small engine for the dinghy that I can work by myself! He knows how much I have missed my "free me" time in the dinghy, birding and exploring early in the morning. YAHOO!! I was really surprised and so very, very excited. Dear Glenn knows how much it means to me to be more independent. How typically thoughtful and sweet of him.

Inspired by a tranquil, rosy-hued sunrise, I decided to take off on a dawn bird patrol and drift in a lovely treelined creek. In this awesome Chesapeake "chapel," I planned to write poetry, read my Bible, swim, and pray. I love floating in the cool green embrace of the Chesapeake, looking up at the scrubbed blue sky and praying, Hi, God, it's me again.

After the pain pills kicked in and I could move, I loaded up the dinghy.

Five pulls on the engine and barroom, I was off on an adventure, zooming down the river at predawn; there was solitude and a warm wind was hugging me. It was exhilarating.

Slowly motoring into the creek, the tree line beckoned me closer where I hoped to see a hawk or perhaps an eagle. I picked up the binoculars scanning the treetops and marshy shore.

The unmistakable cry of a hawk being chased by chattering crows led me down the right branch of the creek. The morning mist swirling along the inky dark water gave me a primeval feeling as I headed down around the bend. When the engine started churning up black mud, I pulled it up, locked it in place, and Huck Finned it with oars to explore the marshy shallow.

Herons were gliding in front of me with barely a flap of their huge gray wings as they flew to the nearby shore, landing soundlessly on their long stilted legs.

Three ospreys were circling high above me. Mom and Pop were mewing to Junior, teaching him the fine art of diving for fish.

I had a front-row seat to savor this dawn of a new day. After spending a couple of hours experiencing some breathtaking sights, the sun was getting higher and hotter and ready to cook this airless cove. I rowed reluctantly away, awash in the serenity and beauty of this never-to-be-forgotten ballet at dawn.

Out deep enough now, it was time to put the engine down and head back to Freyja, but the damn thing had locked solidly and stubbornly in the up position. I pulled, yanked, performed Houdini maneuvers, hit, screamed, and pleaded, but to no avail. I got so angry I was crying. How dare this inanimate thing not bow to my will! If a sledgehammer had been handy, I would joyously have smashed it.

It was a good two miles back to Freyja against the current. What a mess I was in. Here I was in

*the middle of nowhere, and Freyja was not even
in sight.*

*Luckily I had a water jug aboard so I calmed
myself down and began the long row home.*

Annie always enjoyed being able to relive both her
good and bad experiences with Glenn, which she related
so vividly that he could share them almost like he had been
there with her. I love that Annie, in spite of her closeness
with Glenn, was also independent enough to enjoy her own
adventures and time to herself. They thoroughly enjoyed
being with each other but were not so codependent that
they didn't also appreciate their own space. Their own
individual experiences gave them food for conversation,
making their time together even more special.

*A chorus of tree frogs and locusts started their
evening serenade around 9:00 as we finished a
steak dinner with salad and fresh corn. It was a
spectacular star-studded night. All around us was
just so incredibly serene and breathtaking. I shall
never forget how happy and secure I felt with my
precious Glenn by my side, sharing the splendor and
sheer joy of the evening. Beauty shared is always
doubly appreciated.*

*The unerring constancy, beauty, and mystery
of God's universe remains year in and year out. It
matters little what happens in our small lives. We're
just a speck, barely a pinpoint, in the gargantuan
scheme of nature, which is both comforting and*

humbling. I find comfort in knowing that the sea will always roll on, changing tides. There will always be a sunrise, sunset, new moon, and full moon as the cycle of life continues. Our time on this earth is so brief. My reward is being healthy enough to enjoy this gift of a world we inhabit.

I have read in Annie's journals where she would end such a passage by laughing at herself with a self-conscious remark, such as "Good heavens, I hope no one ever reads this Pollyanna babble, but God has blessed me so that sometimes I want to hug the heavens." But I certainly never felt that it was Pollyanna babble and always enjoyed the combination of reverence, appreciation, and joy with which Annie greeted the universe. I also loved her insightful perceptions.

All of October has passed and November has a bite out of it with each sunny day threatening to be the last. One more rain storm and the final, tenacious leaves will release their precarious hold on their life source and proceed to continue in the eternal dance of life as they float to the woods' floor. Their decaying will provide nourishment and protection to life developing beneath them in the hardening earth. Seeds, resting warm, protected and nourished by the leaves will be ready to burst forth in the coming spring.

Leaves are twirling and floating in a downward spiral to their final resting spot on the woods' floor where they will nourish and maintain the soil and offer a hiding place beneath.

There are many that are floating on the pond's surface, and when they become waterlogged they sink and become shelter for burrowing turtles and bull frogs and feed the pond soil, creating food for aquatic insects. And all of this comes from a rather simple, ordinary dead leaf.

I think that my leaf is getting ready to release its grip on its life-sustaining branch. I shall take time to dance with the wind, float, flutter, and take a twirl or two for exuberance as I spiral down to earth, dead, separate from my life source tree.

But what does dead mean? As the leaf breaks down, it nourishes the earth and aquatic or land bugs. Leaves provide a shelter, a cover on the dirt floor of the woods forming a carpet with other dead leaves, protecting and nourishing new growth beneath them that is waiting to burst forth in springtime. So are leaves more valuable on the tree or after they die?

Can I, will I have done anything that will enable my death to be a healing, nourishing, and protective event? Nothing can ever truly die. Matter cannot be completely destroyed. Nothing ever dies without leaving a trace.

Annie, your death left more than a trace in the lives of everyone who knew you, and not only was your death "healing, nourishing, and protective," but your life was as well—so bursting with experiences. As your biographer, I have had to make selections for our book—when as your sister and friend, I would have chosen to leave in everything! One more story for this chapter:

> We decided to go ashore and walk up to the high bank overlooking the base of the cove. Tippy was scampering joyously ahead of us, his whole body wagging excitedly. We stopped and then moved slowly forward to the edge of the bluff overlooking the water. Hundreds of geese were swimming about looking like a floating island.
>
> And then, we heard, no felt a mighty whoosh, and flying by so close to us, eye-to-eye, was a full grown bald eagle, his white hood gleaming in the setting sun with golden talons tucked toward his massive dark belly. Using his fully fanned white tail as a rudder, he flew sideways close to the tree line. His massive black wings were spread to their full six-foot span. But it was his eyes that pierced right through my being, yellow, glinting sparks, looking right at us. I felt as though I could reach out and touch him. Such closeness. His power was palpable, and his grace and majesty literally stole my breath. Emotions swirled; tangled joy, wonder, amazement. With mouths agape, neither of us spoke, just gripped our hands more tightly. We did not talk or move, not wanting to spoil the magic. Did that actually happen? So close and high up with him, sharing his domain. In a sudden encounter, in a speck of time, we felt the wings of an eagle.

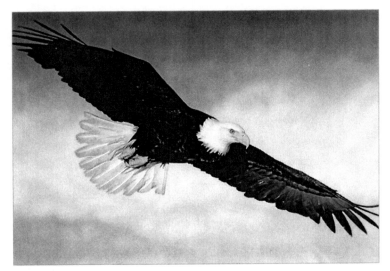

"I felt as though I could reach out and touch him."

CHAPTER FOURTEEN

"Hi, God!"

❧

 EELING ANNIE'S GUIDANCE I considered ending this book with a symbolic gesture that she insisted on doing that left the rest of us in awe and disbelief.

I don't know when the tradition started, and only Annie would be crazy enough to even attempt it, but every New Year's Day, if she wasn't in the hospital or totally incapacitated, Glenn, succumbing to her will, would drive Annie to Stone Harbor and take a photo of her doing a perfect handstand on the beach in celebration of a year past and a new year just beginning.

It still amazes me how she was capable of doing this acrobatic skill in spite of all of her serious and debilitating health problems, but nevertheless, her muscles were strong and she was able to do a nice handstand for many years.

Then once more Annie's voice spoke to me, reminding me of how much she loved to sing. It was another way that she could express herself, and her emotions would explode into song. Annie's enthusiasm for singing exceeded her talent, but that never stopped her.

Annie wanted so much to be in the choir at Marjorie Webster Junior College in Washington, DC. She had such desire and tried so hard that the director let her in with the stipulation that she would just mouth the words. The director said, "I have never known anyone who wanted to sing so badly . . . and did."

Annie delighted in singing hymns with her father, who had a glorious, booming baritone voice. One of my warmest memories was when Annie, her father, Gramma, and I sang a few old hymn favorites with great joy and reverence. We were gathered in the family room of Pops's old historic farmhouse, and I was aware that I was participating in a very special time.

Philip, Annie's father, had grown up singing hymns with his mother and this tradition was passed on to his two daughters. Tyler inherited her father's ability to sing but Annie just inherited the love. Other than hymns, her father's favorite song to perform for anyone who would listen was "Old Man River."

Annie always had a special Christmas message on her answering machine that would amuse any caller. It was different every year but my favorite was her singing parody to the tune of "Jingle Bells." The words were cleverly rhymed and the tune was actually distinguishable. At one point she interrupted herself to mumble, "Oh, now where did I put those bells . . . oh yes," and then you heard a giggle and the jingle of bells.

Living in a suburb outside of Philadelphia, I was able to spend more time with Annie when she was hospitalized in Philadelphia than when she was home in New Jersey. These were also the times when she needed the most support. During one of my visits, a nurse told me that the day before, from far down the hall, she heard someone singing "The Star Spangled Banner" at the top of their lungs. Seeking out the patriotic patient, she found Annie belting out the national anthem with the soloist before the start of a ball game.

Friends or family who sailed with Annie and Glenn were occasionally awakened at 5:30 or so in the morning by Annie, who was greeting the day with a song from the cockpit, and it seemed that Annie didn't know how to sing quietly.

Knowing that Annie would want her life story to end on a high, the perfect anecdote came to me quickly as if she had just whispered in my ear, and suddenly I knew what would make her happy. It's as if she were saying to me that this is the story to end the book with. This is the one and I agreed.

We had a memorable start to our last hurrah weekend of the summer. Glenn and I along with our friends, Pat and Jim, went parasailing last night! Feelings and sights floating 3,600 feet up in the air defy adequate words!

After I had made the reservations, we met on Jim and Pat's new boat around 4:30. We had happy hour aboard—"Cocktail Courage" summoned with rum punches. Glenn kept saying, "I can't believe I let you talk me into this." I was taut as a high wire anticipating the ride. Heavens, what had I done? I was dressed in my clown outfit for the occasion, screaming yellow and pink tie-dyed overalls.

I had arranged for us to be picked up in the anchorage. It was a cool, clear evening as we zoomed off to the ocean in a neon green speedboat. Glenn was still saying he wasn't going up but would take pictures. Pat was chewing her nails with memories of a horrific white water rafting trip that kept haunting her.

We chose to "fly" over Cape May. It was decided that I would go first to "test" the wind because I was the lightest. And then, before I even had time to think about it, I was hooked up in the harness before I could blink! I stepped onto the aft platform, the boat picked up speed, and with a mighty whoosh I was airborne. Swallowing hard I had to remind myself to breathe. A brilliant yellow-and-orange striped chute billowed above me. There I was, floating over a dark sea with sea gulls flying under me! Up up up I went, looking over Cape May toward a glistening bay. The town below was like a train set with miniature houses, streets, and green tufted trees. The view was breathtaking and then a gust of wind carried me even higher. I could see over to the anchorage with the boats looking like small dots. The panorama was vast, beautiful, awesome, and incredible! The sun was sparkling on the water, the sky was azure blue, and tufts of white clouds were stroking the heavens. "Hi, God!"

The boat was circling below me in ever-widening circles as I drifted and swooped, swirling higher still, with my feet dangling over a moving dark canvas of the ocean. I looked hopefully for dolphins. Joy flooded through me. I was waving and shouting with uncontainable glee and exhilaration, and then I was lowered slowly until my feet brushed through the cool water and then I was up again, up and up. Once more there was a vista of Cape May. It was very quiet except for brief bursts of sound from the motorboat that was carried off in the wind. The huge Christian Admiral Hotel was a mere spot on the shore.

I close my eyes now to try and re-create what I saw and felt. Now I know what is meant by "bird's eye view." The creaking of the canvas straps on the harness made me gulp a few times, but I was too overwhelmed by the beauty to be afraid. I didn't want it to end, but then I was floating down to the boat, gazing about me to absorb, to remember as my heart was pumping in my ears. What an adrenaline rush it had been up there!

I landed easily and was unhooked before I knew what was happening. I went around laughing and hugging the bemused crew who had become slightly bored with it all after a long summer. They responded with smiles and a shake of their heads. Bubbling, I hugged dear Glenn, who said simply,

"I'm going up." Pat was next, eyes aglow, and smiling from ear to ear, buoyed and relaxed after cocktails. Zoom, off she went with the yellow-and-orange parachute billowing behind her, then thunk, it filled with air and up she went. She loved it. Jim went next. All of us were taking pictures. He swung happily up, up, and away. He commented, *"I didn't realize Cape May was so narrow."*

My heart was thumping with gladness that Glenn was going up. As he was muttering, *"I hate heights,"* off he went. He kept looking up at the chute, checking knots I guess. I snapped off the last few pictures as he soared heavenward. Darn, he shot so many of me up there, there was only a few left for his adventure. He loved it!

We were all babbling excitedly a mile a minute as the sun was beginning to set and we were zooming back to our boat.

To give ourselves time to absorb our great adventure, we decided to sail out to watch the sunset. It was a lovely sail out on the ocean as the red ball sun plopped behind the horizon of Cape May. The lighthouse was silhouetted on the distant point, a wonderful sight as the lights of Cape May and Wildwood flashed on a dark shore.

Their boat was a smooth, comfortable sailor. We passed the Yankee schooner in the inlet and also passed the Grey Poupon, which set off its cannon to salute us.

I was so very glad we sailed out on the ocean. It removed that tiny thread of intimidation I felt about sunset sails. Now I'm thinking that it's not too late to do it a lot in September, just grab a hoagie and go.

We motor sailed into the inlet as the blackness of evening settled in. The lights on the shore were confusing, but Pat was a good helmsman. We topped off the evening with a wonderful dinner at the Lobster House.

Whenever times get tough and they inevitably do, I shall close my eyes and drift up and up, visualizing the vast, sparkling ocean, the patchwork scene of Cape May in miniature, the azure blue sky, the panorama, humbling and exhilarating. I shall always remember the night I touched the heavens. Thank you, Lord.

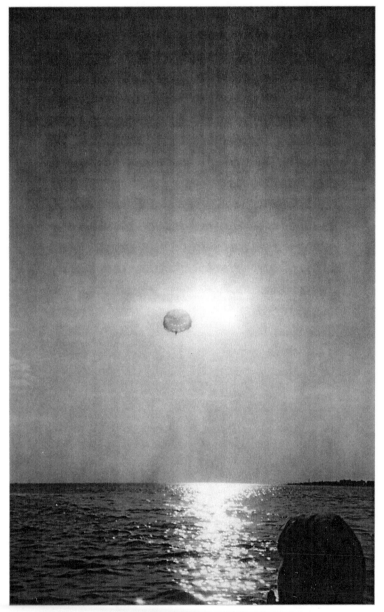

The night Annie touched the heavens

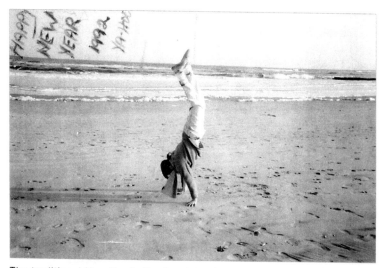

The traditional New Year's Day handstand on the beach

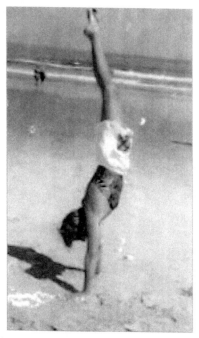

Perfect handstand on the beach in the summer

Acknowledgments

*M*ANY PEOPLE NEED TO BE thanked because for me it would have been next to impossible to complete this book without help. First, I am thankful for Annie who lived such a courageous and adventurous life that needed to be shared. It truly felt as if she were my coauthor, even posthumously, in getting her message out. Then of course there is Glenn who kept her alive with their love for one another and the care he gave her. I appreciate the countless hours you spent with me sharing stories of your lives together.

I also need to thank my dear friend Julie Hunsberger who from the very beginning encouraged me to follow my dream and write the story of Annie's life. Thank you, Julie.

Ralph Stephens, thank you my friend, for being my first reader even before my final draft. I enjoyed our discussions and appreciated your suggestions. It was rewarding to hear how much you loved and believed in *On Eagle's Wings*.

To my friend, John McClay, who fell in love with Annie and offered his professional knowledge of English with proofreading and valuable wording suggestions. Thank you. I have enjoyed our communications and working together to find just the right words.

Much appreciation goes to Dr. Ray Tobey, my friend and advisor to ensure that all medical terms were being correctly used.

My love is always there for my wonderful husband, Ray, who was supportive of my many trips to the cabin in New Jersey, hours and hours talking with Glenn on the phone, card tables sprawled with papers of Annie's life, and spending so much time on my computer for several years. And I am blessed with my son and daughter, David and Lynnie, who are lovingly always there for me in so many ways. They understood how important writing about Annie's life was for all of us who cherish her memory and continue to love her so dearly.

I sincerely thank the wonderful people who willingly agreed to endorse *On Eagle's Wings* with their heartfelt words: Rolf Benirschke, Jon Reiner, John Rombeau, John McClay, Linda Heller, Ray Tobey, Ralph Stephens, Stacey Morgan, Harriet Millan and Laura Sarasqueta.

From 1106 Designs, thank you Ronda, project manager for your friendly efficiency and Laura, proofreader extraordinaire, and the talented cover and interior design department. You were all wonderful to work with.

There is one extremely important person who came into my life as my editor and friend: Stuart Horwitz. He helped me improve the format and realize that revision is largely the art of omission. We worked together with respect, honesty, and humor to find what pleased both of us. Once the writing was completed, he then turned me over to his wonderful associate, Chloe Marsala. Chloe, you were such a pleasure to work with, navigating me through all the decisions that transformed a lot of words into an actual book. You are a gem. Thank you, Stu and Chloe, with all my heart, and I hope that we remain friends forever. By the way, Stuart has written an excellent book on how to write a book called *Blueprint Your Best Seller.*

And finally, I would like to thank everyone who reads *On Eagle's Wings,* hoping that Annie will be an inspiration for you.

About the Author

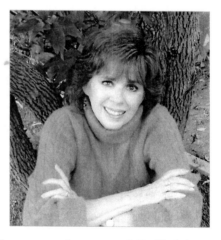

GAIL PARKER always enjoyed writing but never imagined she would end up writing a book. She realized Annie's life story simply needed to be told and spent five years collecting memories and working on the manuscript that became this book. Theater and music have been a major part of Gail's life—she used to sing and perform professionally. She enjoys working with her hands, as well, so when her entertaining days were over, she began a craft business. One of the many things that Gail and Annie bonded over was their love of animals of all kinds. Gail is happily married with two children, three stepchildren, and six grandchildren. She lives in a suburb of Philadelphia.

CPSIA information can be obtained at www.ICGtesting.com
Printed in the USA
BVOW03s0354220514

354219BV00001B/1/P